Breathe Better Today!

Pulmonary Rehabilitation

Comprehensive Course

David Junga, RRT, PAS

Welcome

Dear Students,

Welcome to the Comprehensive Pulmonary Rehabilitation Course Workbook. This workbook is intended to be used side-by-side with your Comprehensive Pulmonary Rehabilitation Online Course. I highly suggest that you print this workbook so that you can fill it in during each lesson. If you don't have access to a printer, I recommend that you have a dedicated notebook for this course to record your answers to the exercises in this workbook.

Taking the time to complete the activities in this workbook is critical for success in this course. Specifically, this workbook takes what would be passive learning and makes it active learning - it forces you to maximize the material being taught through note-taking, investigation, and reflection. Active learning is crucial as it is scientifically proven that this type of learning is correlated with better student engagement, enhanced performance, and increased retention of information.

You can expect to find an overview of the course contained in the table of contents at the beginning of this workbook. Additionally, you will find worksheets for each lesson within the course containing course objectives, goals, to-do lists, and respective assignments. It doesn't take long to complete the workbook but I promise you it will make all the difference in your success!

Sincerely,

David Junga

David Junga, RRT, PAS

Table of Contents

Welcome

Section 1

Section 2

Table of Contents

Section 3

Section 4

Table of Contents

Section 5

Conclusion

Medical & Health Disclaimer

Therapy Programs & Courses
Medical & Health Disclaimer

Information or exercise plans introduced through participation in any of our therapy programs and courses is not a substitute for direct, personal, professional medical care and diagnosis. None of the lifestyle changes, exercises or therapies (including products and services) discussed or utilized in participation with our programs or courses should be performed or otherwise used without clearance from your physician or health care provider.

Section 1

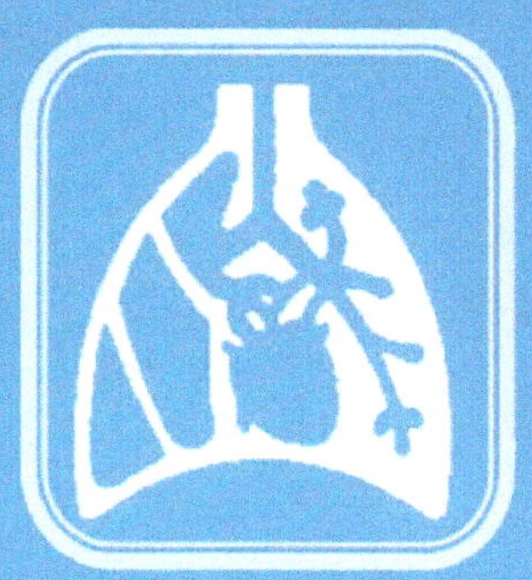

THOUGHT OF THE DAY...

IF YOU DON'T MAKE TIME FOR YOUR *wellness* THEN YOU WILL BE FORCED TO MAKE TIME FOR YOUR *illness.*

LESSON 1: MEET DAVID

Objectives:

I. Familiarize yourself with who David, program director of Pulmonary Rehabilitation Associates, LLC is and his credentials.

II. Understand why Pulmonary Rehabilitation Associates, LLC is different from other Pulmonary Rehabilitation programs.

III. Understand the importance of getting clearance from your Doctor before starting the program.

To-Do:

Watch "Meet David" video, take notes below as needed. ☐

Assignment:

Spend 20-30 minutes exploring PulmonaryRehab.com - scroll around, watch some success stories, look at the blog, etc. **Write down 3-5 interesting things you learned from your research below.**

LESSON 2: WHAT IS PULMONARY REHABILITATION

Objectives:

I. Be able to define what Pulmonary Rehabilitation is.

II. Understand why Pulmonary Rehabilitation is effective.

To-Do:

- [ ] Watch "What is Pulmonary Rehabilitation" video, take notes below as needed.
- [ ] Complete the one question quiz following the video.

Assignment:

Go to pulmonaryrehab.com and click on the "Success Stories" section (https://pulmonaryrehab.com/success-stories/) and watch the Patient testimonials to learn how Pulmonary Rehabilitation changed their lives.

Now that you have heard how Pulmonary Rehabilitation has changed other people's lives, how do you feel Pulmonary Rehabilitation can improve your life? **Please write your response below.**

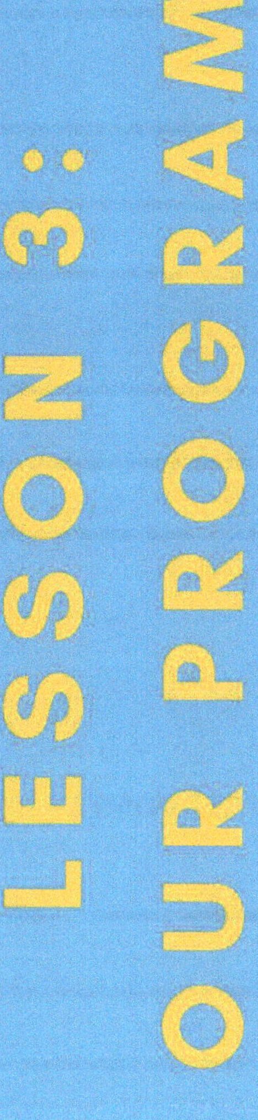

Objectives:

I. Understand and be able to list two reasons why Pulmonary Rehabilitation Associates, LLC is different from all other programs.

II. Be able to define Posture Therapy.

III. Understand the connection between unbalanced posture and shortness of breath.

IV. Be able to define the mind, body, spirit model used in this program.

To-Do:

- [ ] Watch "Our Program" video, take notes below as needed.
- [ ] Complete the one question quiz following the video.

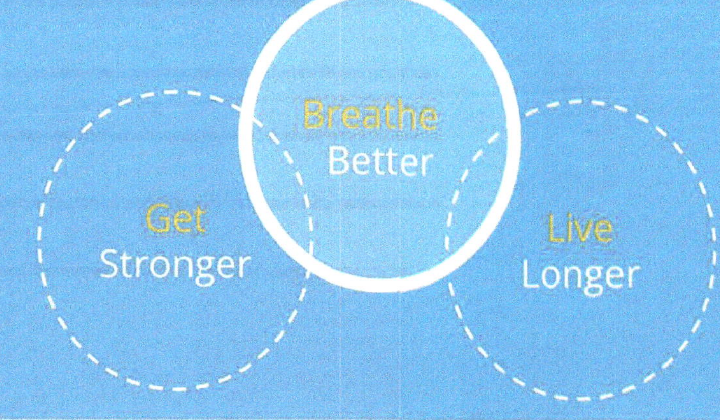

LESSON 3:
OUR PROGRAM

Assignment:

Take 5-10 minutes to reflect on and **write down** what your top 3 goals are for yourself in starting this program.

1

2

3

Keeping these goals in mind, how do you feel as though the Mind Body Spirit model utilized in this program will help you achieve these goals? **Please write your response below.**

LESSON 4: WHO IS THIS PROGRAM FOR

Objective:

I. Understand who this program is designed for.

To-Do:

Watch "Who is this Program For" video, take notes below as needed. ☐

Complete the one question quiz following this video. ☐

Assignment:

Motivation is key for success in this program. Take a few minutes and reflect on what your motivation is to start this program and **write it down below**. Keep this motivation in the back of your mind during this whole program, even consider flipping back to this page every so often for a reminder!

LESSON 5: WHY PULM. REHAB. IS THE MISSING PIECE OF THE PUZZLE

Objectives:

I. Understand why Pulmonary Rehabilitation plays a significant role in the treatment of pulmonary conditions.

II. Understand why exercise is so important for Patients with pulmonary conditions.

To-Do:

- [ ] Watch "Why Pulmonary Rehabilitation is the Missing Piece of the Puzzle" video, take notes below as needed.
- [ ] Complete the one question quiz following the video.

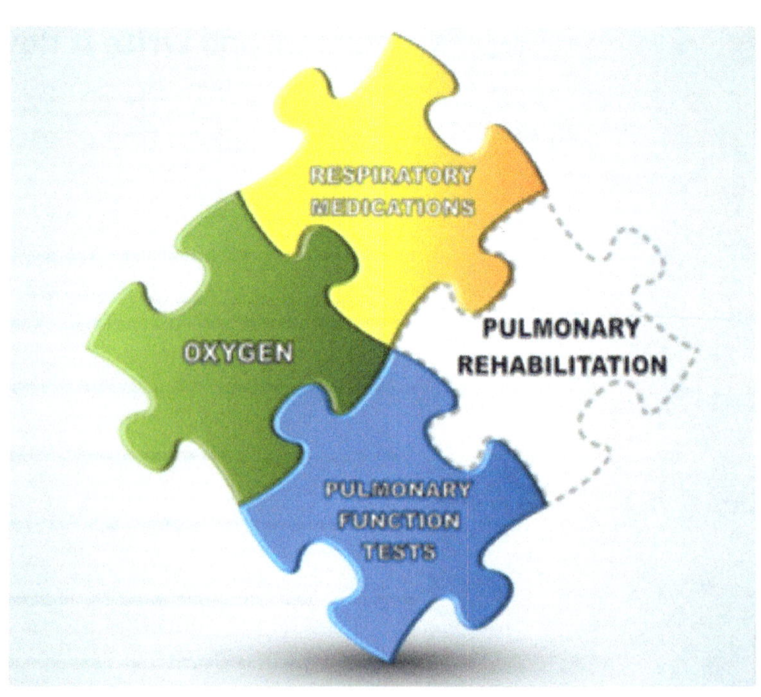

LESSON 5: WHY PULM. REHAB. IS THE MISSING PIECE OF THE PUZZLE

Assignment:

Referencing the image on the previous page, write out what this puzzle looks like for you--are you on oxygen? Respiratory medications? What were your pulmonary function tests? Reflect on the responses to these items; do you want to lessen your medications, lessen your oxygen, etc.? Use this as motivation for this course and **write your response below.**

LESSON 6: HOW DO PULM. REHABILITATION EXERCISES HELP

Objective:

I. Understand the two main reasons why Pulmonary Rehabilitation exercises help reduce your shortness of breath.

To-Do:

- [ ] Watch "How do Pulmonary Rehabilitation Exercises Help" video, take notes below as needed.
- [ ] Complete the one question quiz following the video.

Assignment:

Understanding why Pulmonary Rehabilitation exercises help, list 3 activities that you plan on doing once you are stronger and have less shortness of breath. **Please write your response below.**

1.

2.

3.

LESSON 7: GET YOUR SAFE NUMBERS FROM YOUR DOCTOR

Objective:

I. Understand the importance of speaking with your doctor prior to this program to get your safe range of numbers for your oxygen saturation, heart rate, blood pressure, and respiratory rate.

II. Understand the importance of being an active member in your healthcare team, including having open communication with your providers and asking questions.

To-Do:

- [ ] Watch "Get Your Safe Numbers From Your Doctor" video, take notes below as needed.
- [ ] Complete the one question quiz following this video.

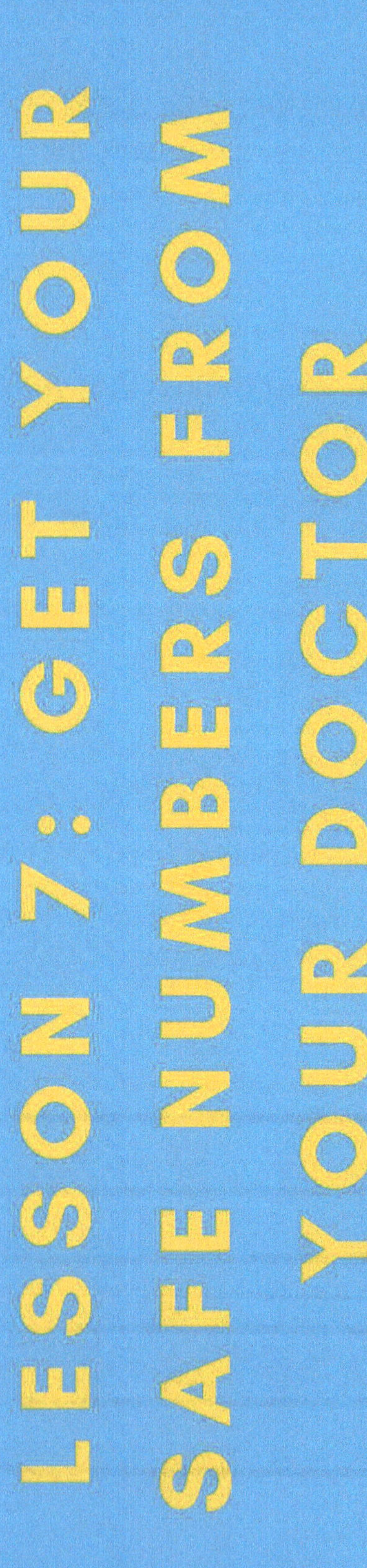

Assignment:

Motivation is key for success in this program. Take a few minutes and reflect on what your motivation is to start this program and **write it down below**. Keep this motivation in the back of your mind during this whole program, even consider flipping back to this page every so often for a reminder!

Section 2

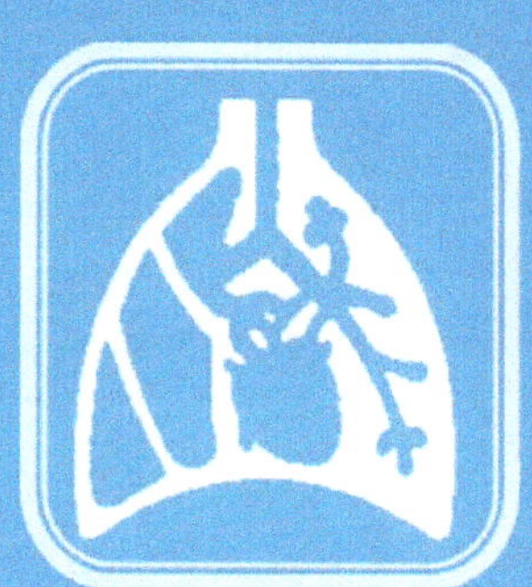

THOUGHT OF THE DAY...

DON'T LET HOW YOU *feel* MAKE YOU FORGET WHAT YOU *deserve.*

LESSON 1: WHAT, HOW, WHEN, WHY TO USE A PULSE OXIMETER

Objectives:

I. Understand the importance of using a pulse oximeter during this course and throughout your day-to-day activities.

II. Use the **Daily Activities Log** to capture your oxygen saturation and heart rate during day-to-day activities.

To-Do:

Watch the "What, How, When, Why to Use a Pulse Oximeter" video, take notes below as needed. ☐

Assignment:

Take some time to familiarize yourself with your pulse oximeter and fill out the **Daily Activities Log** on the following page.

After completing the log, please write below which activities gave you the most difficulty.

- Were you surprised at which activities were challenging?
- Which activities were easy and was this surprising?
- Did your shortness of breath and your oxygen saturation/heart rate match or was your oxygen saturation lower than you expected and your heart rate higher?

LESSON 1: INTRODUCTION TO THE DAILY ACTIVITIES LOG

To-Do:

Watch the "Introduction to the Daily Activities Log" video. ☐

Use the log below to record your lowest oxygen saturation and highest heart rate doing each respective activity. If needed, please refer to the "Introduction to the Daily Activities Log" located in this lesson for a refresher on what this form is and how to use it.

Please circle any oxygen saturation below 92%.

Activity	Date	Time	Lowest Oxygen Sat (%)	Highest Heart Rate (bpm)	Notes
Making the bed					
Showering					
Putting away the groceries					
Doing the dishes					
Vacuuming					
Getting the mail					
Walking the dog					
Emptying the garbage					
Doing the laundry/ironing					
Cooking					
Other					

LESSON 2: INTRODUCTION TO SELF-ASSESSMENTS

Objectives:

I. Understand the purpose and contents of the Self-Assessments in this course.

II. Understand the importance and benefits of tracking your progress using the Self-Assessments in this course.

III. Understand how to use the Self-Assessments in this course.

To-Do:

Watch the "Introduction to Self-Assessments" video, take notes below as needed. ☐

Assignment:

In understanding what the Self-Assessments are, their contents, and how to use them, please list the ways they will be a beneficial tool for you in this course. **Please write your response below.**

LESSON 2: INTRODUCTION TO SELF-ASSESSMENT #1

Objectives:

I. Understand the purpose and contents of **Self-Assessment #1**.

II. Understand how to use **Self-Assessment #1**.

To-Do:

Watch the "Introduction to Self-Assessment #1" video, take notes below as needed. ☐

Assignment:

Before continuing on to complete **Self-Assessment #1**, please take some time to continue to familiarize yourself with **Self-Assessment #1** by flipping through the next 7 pages in this workbook. Take notes below as needed.

LESSON 2: SELF-ASSESSMENT #1

CAPTURING AND RECORDING YOUR INITIAL NUMBERS: AT REST & EXERCISING

Objectives:

I. Offers a baseline assessment of your oxygen saturation and heart rate at rest and while exercising.

II. Allows for reflection on the current state of your lungs, heart, and your breathing and provides an opportunity to identify future health goals.

III. Provides a reference point when comparing oxygen saturation and heart rate at the beginning of the program in comparison to other checkpoints throughout the program to quantify your progress.

To-Do:

After listening to the explanation of what the self-assessment is and the importance of it, while ***at rest***, check and record your oxygen saturation and heart rate below using a pulse oximeter.

As a reminder, put the pulse oximeter on your finger and wait about 20 seconds to allow the device to capture the most accurate readings.

If you find that your oxygen saturation and heart rate readings are much different than your normal readings, please put the device on your other hand, trying multiple fingers until you get the best signal strength and reading.

Repeat this 3 times to get a total of 3 oxygen saturation and heart rate readings, waiting approximately 2 minutes between each reading.

LESSON 2:
SELF-ASSESSMENT #1

CAPTURING AND RECORDING YOUR INITIAL NUMBERS: AT REST & EXERCISING

Pulse Oximeter Reading #1 (AT REST)

Oxygen Saturation (%)	
Heart Rate (bpm)	
Supplemental Oxygen (L) *(if you don't wear oxygen, write "room air")*	

Pulse Oximeter Reading #2 (AT REST)

Oxygen Saturation (%)	
Heart Rate (bpm)	
Supplemental Oxygen (L) *(if you don't wear oxygen, write "room air")*	

Pulse Oximeter Reading #3 (AT REST)

Oxygen Saturation (%)	
Heart Rate (bpm)	
Supplemental Oxygen (L) *(if you don't wear oxygen, write "room air")*	

LESSON 2: SELF-ASSESSMENT #1

CAPTURING AND RECORDING YOUR INITIAL NUMBERS: AT REST & EXERCISING

Reflection:

Take a few minutes and reflect on how your breathing felt while at rest:

- Did you feel short of breath?
- Did you breathe through your nose, mouth, or a combination of both?
- Did you experience any coughing or wheezing?

Record any other notable observations. My goal is for you to be able to predict what your oxygen saturation and heart rate are based on how you feel.

Please don't let the pulse oximeter dictate how you feel!

Please record your responses to the above questions in the space below.

LESSON 2: SELF-ASSESSMENT #1

CAPTURING AND RECORDING YOUR INITIAL NUMBERS: AT REST & EXERCISING

To-Do:

Now, we want to capture what your oxygen saturation and heart rate are ***during exercise.*** **Choose whether you would like to walk in place for 1 minute or walk down a hallway for 1 minute - choose whichever you are more comfortable with.** Be sure to have your pulse oximeter on your finger and to set a timer for 1 minute. If you find that 1 minute is too long, please stop as needed and exercise for whatever length of time is most comfortable for you.

Begin walking in place or down a hallway when you press 'start' on the timer. When the timer goes off, be sure to check and record your oxygen saturation and heart rate below.

As a reminder, put the pulse oximeter on your finger and wait about 20 seconds to allow the device to capture the most accurate readings. If you find that your oxygen saturation and heart rate readings are much different than your normal readings, please put the device on your other hand, trying multiple fingers until you get the best signal strength and reading.

Repeat this 3 times to get a total of 3 oxygen saturation and heart rate readings, waiting approximately 2 minutes or as long as it takes to catch your breath between each reading.

As a reminder, please check your oxygen saturation and heart rate readings frequently during this exercise. If you find that your oxygen saturation drops below or your heart rate goes above the accepted values your healthcare providers gave to you, immediately stop.

Reminder: I usually recommend maintaining an oxygen saturation of 92% or higher.

LESSON 2: SELF-ASSESSMENT #1

CAPTURING AND RECORDING YOUR INITIAL NUMBERS: AT REST & EXERCISING

Pulse Oximeter Reading #1 (exercising)
Circle one: Hallway walking or walking in place

Oxygen Saturation (%)	
Heart Rate (bpm)	
Supplemental Oxygen (L) (if you don't wear oxygen, write "room air")	
Total time walking (min or sec)	
ONLY FOR HALLWAY: Distance (steps, ft, mi)	

Pulse Oximeter Reading #2 (exercising)
Circle one: Hallway walking or walking in place

Oxygen Saturation (%)	
Heart Rate (bpm)	
Supplemental Oxygen (L) (if you don't wear oxygen, write "room air")	
Total time walking (min or sec)	
ONLY FOR HALLWAY: Distance (steps, ft, mi)	

Pulse Oximeter Reading #3 (exercising)
Circle one: Hallway walking or walking in place

Oxygen Saturation (%)	
Heart Rate (bpm)	
Supplemental Oxygen (L) (if you don't wear oxygen, write "room air")	
Total time walking (min or sec)	
ONLY FOR HALLWAY: Distance (steps, ft, mi)	

LESSON 2: SELF-ASSESMENT #1

CAPTURING AND RECORDING YOUR INITIAL NUMBERS: AT REST & EXERCISING

Reflection:

Take a few minutes and reflect on how your breathing felt while exercising (walking):

- Did you feel short of breath?
- Did you have to take any breaks during the 1 minute?
- Did 1 minute feel like a long time?
- How long did it take for you to catch your breath after the 1 minute timer went off?

Please record your responses to the above questions in the space below.

LESSON 2: SELF-ASSESSMENT #1

CAPTURING AND RECORDING YOUR INITIAL NUMBERS: AT REST & EXERCISING

Reflection:

Reflect on your experience with the previous two activities:

- Were you surprised at your oxygen saturation and heart rate values?
- Did you find these activities challenging?
- What are some current obstacles you feel with your breathing that you hope this program will help you overcome?

Please record your responses to the above questions in the space below.

Great job! You've completed your initial assessment! Make sure that all the above information is filled out and keep this assessment in a safe place, you will need to reference it later on in the course.

LESSON 3: WHY ARE YOUR SHORT OF BREATH

Objectives:

I. Understand the Shortness of Breath Cycle.

II. Identify the two main causes of pulmonary related shortness of breath.

To-Do:

- [ ] Watch "Why are you short of breath" video, take notes below as needed.
- [ ] Complete the one question quiz following this video

Assignment:

Reflect on the Shortness of Breath Cycle introduced in the earlier video. Does this sound familiar to you? How has shortness of breath impacted your life and the lives of your loved ones? **Please write your response below.**

LESSON 4: INTRO. TO THE SHORTNESS OF BREATH SCALE

Objectives:

I. Understand the purpose of the **Shortness of Breath Scale** and how to use it to quantify your shortness of breath.

II. Use the **Shortness of Breath Scale** to get a baseline quantification of your shortness of breath.

To-Do:

Watch the "Introduction to the Shortness of Breath Scale" video, take notes below as needed. ☐

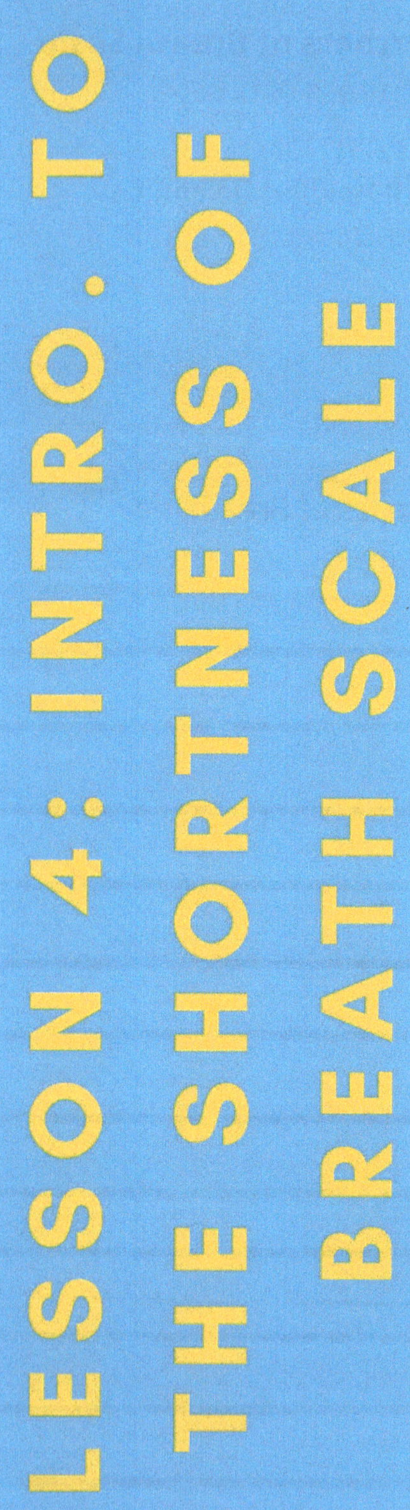

Use the **Shortness of Breath Scale** below to quantify your shortness of breath by circling the column containing the SOB number that best describes how you feel.

***If you need a refresher on what this scale is and how to use it, please reference the video earlier in this lesson called "Introduction to the Shortness of Breath Scale".*

SOB #	0	½	1	2	3	4	5	6	7	8
SEVERITY	NONE	JUST NOTICEABLE	VERY SLIGHT	SLIGHT	MODERATE	MORE MODERATE	SEVERE	MORE SEVERE	VERY SEVERE	MAXIMUM
	Normal Speech				Choppy Speech		Can't Speak		Call 911!	

LESSON 5: POSTURE AND BREATHING: HOW ARE THEY RELATED

Objective:

1. Understand the two main ways poor posture can contribute to shortness of breath.

To-Do:

- [ ] Watch the "Posture and Breathing: How are They Related" video, take notes below as needed.
- [ ] Complete the one question quiz following the video.

Assignment:

Look at your posture in a mirror. Are your shoulders or upper back rounded forward? Is your head forward? Are your feet either duck-footed or pigeon-toed? How do you think your posture is impacting your breathing? **Please write your response below.**

Section 3

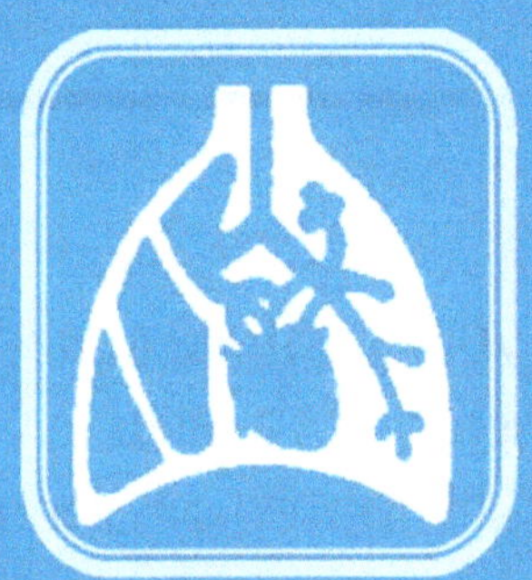

THOUGHT OF THE DAY...

YOUR *speed*
DOESN'T MATTER,
PROGRESS IS
progress AND
FORWARD IS
forward.

LESSON 1: FLOW-CONTROLLED BREATHING©

Objectives:

I. Understand why forced exhalation isn't effective.

II. Understand the 3 distinct phases of Flow-Controlled Breathing©, including the importance of the "hold" phase.

III. Understand why taking a normal sized breath in through your nose is most effective.

IV. Understand how long you need to breathe in and blow out while doing Flow-Controlled Breathing©.

To-Do:

- [ ] Read about what Flow-Controlled Breathing© is and how it works, take notes below as needed.

REQUIRED MATERIALS

- PULSE OXIMETER
- SUPPLEMENTAL OXYGEN, IF PRESCRIBED
- TISSUE OR NAPKIN

LESSON 1: FLOW-CONTROLLED BREATHING©

To-Do:

- [ ] Watch the "Flow Controlled Breathing©: A Step-By-Step Guide" video, take notes below as needed.
- [ ] Complete the one question quiz following this video.

___

___

___

___

___

Assignment:

Now that you have learned about Flow-Controlled Breathing©, please take this time to practice this new breathing method now and daily until you can do it on demand.

Use **Self-Assessment #2**, beginning on **page 34**, while practicing

LESSON 2: INTRODUCTION TO SELF-ASSESSMENT #2

Objectives:

I. Understand the purpose and contents of **Self-Assessment #2**.

II. Understand how to use **Self-Assessment #2**.

To-Do:

Watch the "Introduction to Self-Assessment #2" video, take notes below as needed. ☐

Assignment:

Before continuing on to complete **Self-Assessment #2**, please take some time to continue to familiarize yourself with **Self-Assessment #2** by flipping through the next 5 pages in this workbook. Take notes below as needed.

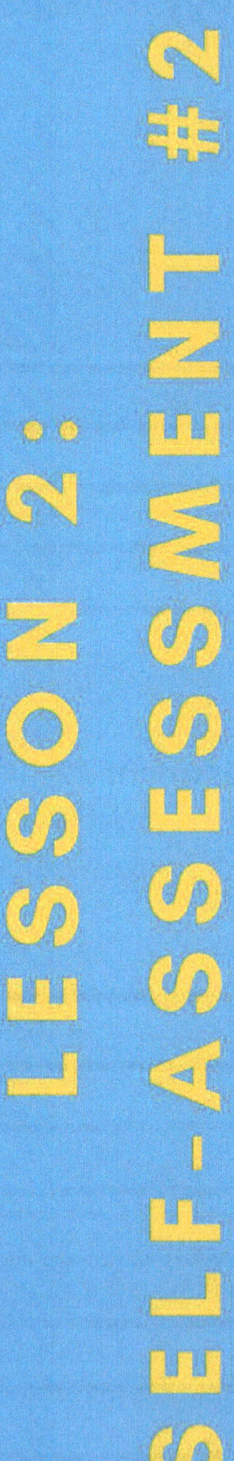

CAPTURING AND RECORDING YOUR INITIAL NUMBERS: PRACTICING FLOW-CONTROLLED BREATHING©

Objectives:

I. Provides an opportunity to compare oxygen saturation and heart rate without using the Flow-Controlled Breathing© technique vs. using the Flow-Controlled Breathing© technique.

II. Allows a reference point when comparing oxygen saturation and heart rate at this point in the program in comparison to other checkpoints in the program to quantify your progress.

III. Allows quantification of shortness of breath after doing the Flow-Controlled Breathing© technique using the **Shortness of Breath Scale**.

IV. Provides a quantitative comparison of shortness of breath using the Flow-Controlled Breathing© technique versus not using the Flow-Controlled Breathing© technique.

To-Do:

After watching the Flow-Controlled Breathing© step-by-step guide, while ***at rest***, ***breathe as you normally would*** ***(don't do the Flow-Controlled Breathing© yet!)*** now check and record your oxygen saturation and heart rate on the next page using a pulse oximeter.

As a reminder, put the pulse oximeter on your finger and wait about 20 seconds to allow the device to capture the most accurate readings.

If you find that your oxygen saturation and heart rate readings are much different than your normal readings, please put the device on your other hand, trying multiple fingers until you get the best signal strength and reading.

LESSON 2: SELF-ASSESSMENT #2

CAPTURING AND RECORDING YOUR INITIAL NUMBERS: PRACTICING FLOW-CONTROLLED BREATHING©

Pulse Oximeter Reading (AT REST, normal breathing)

Oxygen Saturation (%)	
Heart Rate (bpm)	
Supplemental Oxygen (L) *(if you don't wear oxygen, write "room air")*	

To-Do:

Wait *2 minutes* after the above reading is taken and then while ***at rest***, **begin the *Flow-Controlled Breathing© technique***, as described in the Flow-Controlled Breathing© step-by-step guide, taking 4-6 Flow-Controlled breaths and check and record your oxygen saturation and heart rate on the next page using a pulse oximeter.

As a reminder, put the pulse oximeter on your finger and wait about 20 seconds to allow the device to capture the most accurate readings.

If you find that your oxygen saturation and heart rate readings are much different than your normal readings, please put the device on your other hand, trying multiple fingers until you get the best signal strength and reading.

LESSON 2:
SELF-ASSESSMENT #2

CAPTURING AND RECORDING YOUR INITIAL NUMBERS: PRACTICING FLOW-CONTROLLED BREATHING©

Pulse Oximeter Reading (AT REST, Flow-Controlled Breathing©)

Oxygen Saturation (%)	
Heart Rate (bpm)	
Supplemental Oxygen (L) *(if you don't wear oxygen, write "room air")*	

Reflection:

Take a few minutes and compare your oxygen saturation and heart rate from normal breathing vs. using the Flow-Controlled Breathing© technique.

- Are both the oxygen saturation and heart rate different?
- How did the Flow-Controlled Breathing© technique feel?
- In doing the Flow-Controlled Breathing© technique, did your breathing feel more smooth?
- Were you less short of breath? Record any other notable observations from the above exercise.

Please record your responses to the above questions in the space below.

LESSON 2: SELF-ASSESSMENT #2

CAPTURING AND RECORDING YOUR INITIAL NUMBERS: PRACTICING FLOW-CONTROLLED BREATHING©

After practicing the Flow-Controlled Breathing© technique, use the **Shortness of Breath Scale** below to quantify your shortness of breath by circling the column containing the shortness of breath number that best describes how you feel.

***If you need a refresher on what this scale is and how to use it, please reference the video in Section 2 Lesson 4 entitled "Introduction to the Shortness of Breath Scale".*

Shortness of Breath Scale

SOB #	0	½	1	2	3	4	5	6	7	8
SEVERITY	NONE	JUST NOTICEABLE	VERY SLIGHT	SLIGHT	MODERATE	MORE MODERATE	SEVERE	MORE SEVERE	VERY SEVERE	MAXIMUM
	Normal Speech				Choppy Speech		Can't Speak		Call 911!	

LESSON 2: SELF-ASSESSMENT #2

CAPTURING AND RECORDING YOUR INITIAL NUMBERS: PRACTICING FLOW-CONTROLLED BREATHING©

Reflection:

Take a few minutes and compare the shortness of breath number you chose above compared to the one you chose back in Section 2, Lesson 4 **(page 26)**. What are the numbers you chose?

Hopefully, you noticed a decrease in your shortness of breath. If you did not, please continue to practice the Flow-Controlled Breathing© technique until you feel an improvement in your shortness of breath.

If you did experience noticeable improvement in your shortness of breath, **congratulations**! Keep up the good work!

Record any other notable observations below.

___

___

___

___

___

___

___

___

Great job, you've completed your second assessment! Make sure that all the information is filled out and keep this assessment in a safe place.

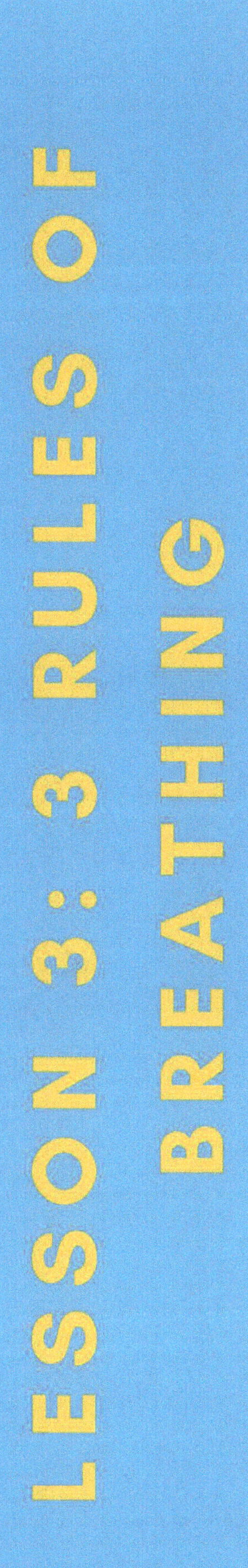

Objective:

I. Understand what the 3 Rules of Breathing are and the importance of using them throughout this course.

To-Do:

- [ ] Watch the "3 Rules of Breathing" video, take notes below as needed.
- [ ] Complete the one question quiz following the video.

Assignment:

Now that you have learned about the 3 Rules of Breathing, please apply them to how you breathe:

- What feels different?
- Do you feel less short of breath?
- Do you feel more balanced?
- Do you feel a reduction in the tension of your shoulders and neck?

Please write your response below.

LESSON 4: WALKING WITH FLOW-CONTROLLED BREATHING©

REQUIRED MATERIALS

- ☑ PULSE OXIMETER
- ☑ SUPPLEMENTAL OXYGEN, IF PRESCRIBED
- ☑ WATER (GLASS OR BOTTLE)

LESSON 4: INTRODUCTION TO THE WORK SCALE

Objective:

I. Understand the purpose of the **Work Scale** and how to use it to quantify the amount of work you do while exercising.

To-Do:

Watch the "Introduction to the Work Scale" video, take notes below as needed. ☐

Assignment:

How do you think quantifying the amount of work you do while exercising could be beneficial? **Please write your response below.**

LESSON 4: WALKING WITH FLOW-CONTROLLED BREATHING©

Objectives:

I. Understand how to combine Flow-Controlled Breathing© with walking.

II. Understand the importance of allowing your breathing to dictate your walking pace, NOT the other way around.

III. Understand the appropriate steps you should take should you get winded while walking.

To-Do:

- [ ] Watch the "Walking with Flow Controlled Breathing©" video, take notes below as needed.
- [ ] Complete the one question quiz following the video.

____

____

____

____

____

Assignment:

Now that you have seen how to incorporate Flow-Controlled Breathing© with walking, take this time to try it out! Use **Self-Assessment #3** beginning on **page 44** while practicing.

Remember, this is the first step--pun intended - to getting better and improving your quality of life, be patient... Each time you do this, you will improve. You've got this!

LESSON 5: INTRODUCTION TO SELF-ASSESSMENT #3

Objectives:

I. Understand the purpose and contents of **Self-Assessment #3**.

II. Understand how to use **Self-Assessment #3**.

To-Do:

Watch the "Introduction to Self-Assessment #3" video, take notes below as needed. ☐

Assignment:

Before continuing on to complete **Self-Assessment #3**, please take some time to continue to familiarize yourself with **Self-Assessment #3** by flipping through the next 8 pages in this workbook. Take notes below as needed.

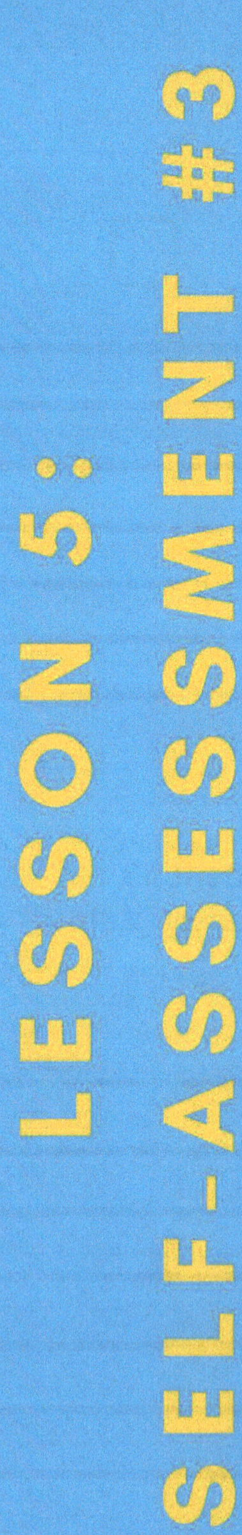

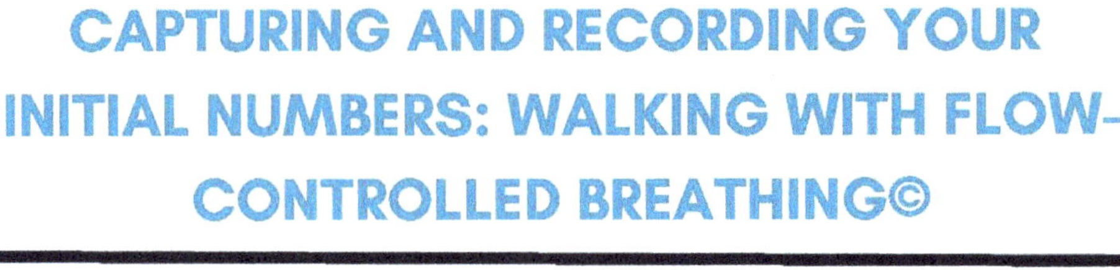

Objectives:

I. Allows practice of walking while utilizing the Flow-Controlled Breathing© technique and an opportunity to reflect on this new way to breath.

II. Provides a reference point when comparing oxygen saturation and heart rate at this point in the program in comparison to other checkpoints in the program to quantify your progress.

III. Provides quantification of shortness of breath after walking with the Flow-Controlled Breathing© technique using the **Shortness of Breath Scale**.

IV. Provides quantification of the amount of work done after walking with the Flow-Controlled Breathing© technique using the **Work Scale**.

To-Do:

Following watching the "Walking with Flow-Controlled Breathing©" video, put your pulse oximeter on your finger and begin walking in a hallway using the Flow-Controlled Breathing© technique explained in the above video.

Be sure to take rests when necessary and check and record your numbers ***before, during, and upon completion*** of walking on the next few pages.

LESSON 5: SELF-ASSESSMENT #3

CAPTURING AND RECORDING YOUR INITIAL NUMBERS: WALKING WITH FLOW-CONTROLLED BREATHING©

To-Do (continued):

Try your best to capture *2-3 oxygen saturation and heart rate readings* from your pulse oximeter ***DURING*** the time you are walking and separate each below in the appropriate box with commas.

As a reminder, put the pulse oximeter on your finger and wait about 20 seconds to allow the device to capture the most accurate readings. If you find that your oxygen saturation and heart rate readings are much different than your normal readings, please put the device on your other hand, trying multiple fingers until you get the best signal strength and reading.

As a reminder, please check your oxygen saturation and heart rate readings frequently during this exercise. If you find that your oxygen saturation drops below or your heart rate goes above the accepted values your healthcare providers gave to you, immediately stop.

Reminder: I usually recommend maintaining an oxygen saturation of 92% or higher.

Pulse Oximeter Reading (Before walking)

Oxygen Saturation (%)	
Heart Rate (bpm)	
Supplemental Oxygen (L) *(if you don't wear oxygen, write "room air")*	

LESSON 5: SELF-ASSESSMENT #3

CAPTURING AND RECORDING YOUR INITIAL NUMBERS: WALKING WITH FLOW-CONTROLLED BREATHING©

Pulse Oximeter Reading
(During walking; multiple readings separated by commas)

Oxygen Saturation (%)	
Heart Rate (bpm)	
Supplemental Oxygen (L) *(if you don't wear oxygen, write "room air")*	
Number of rests	
Distance (steps, ft, mi)	
Total time walking (min)	

Pulse Oximeter Reading (After walking)

Oxygen Saturation (%)	
Heart Rate (bpm)	
Supplemental Oxygen (L) *(if you don't wear oxygen, write "room air")*	

LESSON 5: SELF-ASSESSMENT #3

CAPTURING AND RECORDING YOUR INITIAL NUMBERS: WALKING WITH FLOW-CONTROLLED BREATHING©

To-Do:

After incorporating Flow-Controlled Breathing© with walking, use the **Shortness of Breath Scale** below to quantify your shortness of breath by circling the column containing the shortness of breath number that best describes how you feel.

***If you need a refresher on what this scale is and how to use it, please reference the video in Section 2 Lesson 4 entitled "Introduction to the Shortness of Breath Scale".*

Shortness of Breath Scale

SOB #	0	½	1	2	3	4	5	6	7	8
SEVERITY	NONE	JUST NOTICEABLE	VERY SLIGHT	SLIGHT	MODERATE	MORE MODERATE	SEVERE	MORE SEVERE	VERY SEVERE	MAXIMUM
	Normal Speech				Choppy Speech		Can't Speak		Call 911!	

LESSON 5:
SELF-ASSESSMENT #3

CAPTURING AND RECORDING YOUR INITIAL NUMBERS: WALKING WITH FLOW-CONTROLLED BREATHING©

Reflection:

Take a few minutes and compare the shortness of breath number you chose, compared to how you felt after completing the walking portion of **Self-Assessment #1** (**page 21-23**). What are the numbers you chose?

Hopefully, you noticed a decrease in your shortness of breath. If you did not, please continue to practice incorporating the Flow-Controlled Breathing© technique while walking until you notice an improvement in your shortness of breath.

If you did experience a noticeable improvement in your shortness of breath, **congratulations**! Keep up the good work!

Record any other notable observations below.

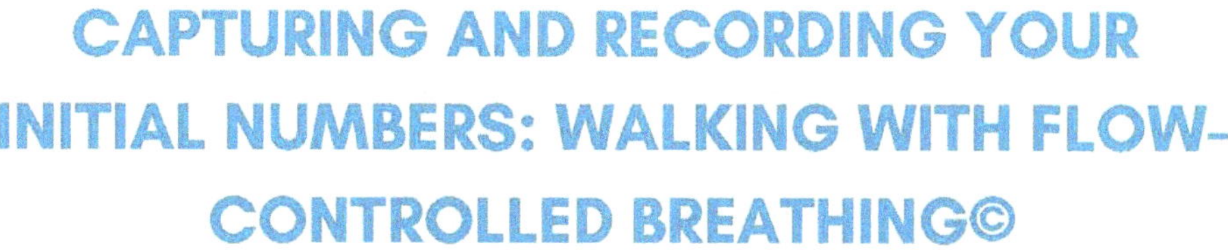

CAPTURING AND RECORDING YOUR INITIAL NUMBERS: WALKING WITH FLOW-CONTROLLED BREATHING©

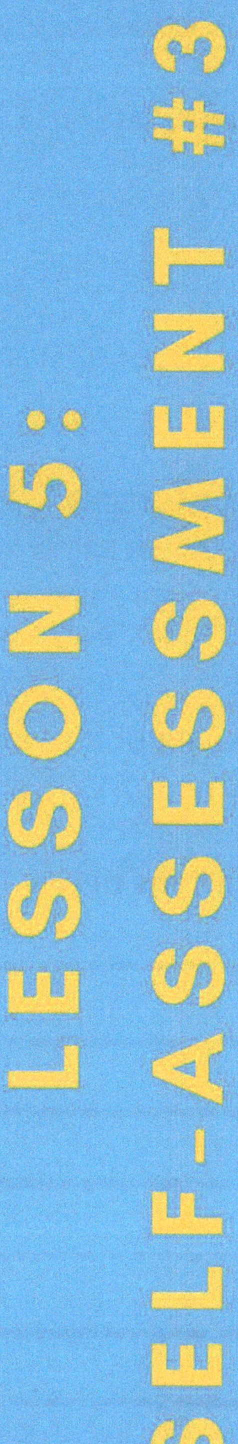

To-Do:

After incorporating Flow-Controlled Breathing© with walking, use the **Work Scale** below to quantify the amount of work you performed during this exercise by circling the column containing the work number that best describes how you feel.

***If you need a refresher on what this scale is and how to use it, please reference the video in Section 3 Lesson 4 entitled "Introduction to the Work Scale".*

How difficult is the exercise that you are doing right now?

This is no work at all	Not bad at all, but too easy	A little harder, but still good	This is good, I'm challenged	Getting too difficult	Nope, can't do it
0	1	2	3	4	5

Let's try and stay between 2 and 3.5

LESSON 5: SELF-ASSESSMENT #3

CAPTURING AND RECORDING YOUR INITIAL NUMBERS: WALKING WITH FLOW-CONTROLLED BREATHING©

Reflection:

Take a few minutes and reflect on the number you chose from the **Work Scale**.

- Was it what you expected?
- Was it higher or lower than you expected?
- If it was not in the ideal **2-3.5 range**, what do you plan to do differently next time?

If the number was above this **2-3.5 range**, by continuing to exercise your muscles will strengthen and you will see a noticeable decrease in the amount of work required to do this same activity.

If you did have a noticeable decrease in the amount of work required, **congratulations**! Keep up the good work!

Record any other notable observations below.

LESSON 5: SELF-ASSESSMENT #3

CAPTURING AND RECORDING YOUR INITIAL NUMBERS: WALKING WITH FLOW-CONTROLLED BREATHING©

Reflection:

- How did walking with Flow-Controlled Breathing© feel?
- What feels different doing the Flow-Controlled Breathing© compared to how you normally breathe and walk?
- How did your oxygen saturation and heart rate compare before, during, and after exercise?
- Did you feel short of breath? If you were short of breath, were you doing Flow-Controlled Breathing©? Were you walking too fast?
- How long did it take you to recover after finishing walking?

Record any other notable observations. Now, compare your oxygen saturation and heart rate during exercise using Flow-Controlled Breathing© vs. your oxygen saturation and heart rate while exercising in your first assessment. What has improved? Can you feel these improvements?

Please record your responses to the above questions in the space below.

___

___

___

___

___

___

Great job, you've completed your third assessment! Make sure that all the above information is filled out and keep this assessment in a safe place.

LESSON 6: FLOW-CONTROLLED BREATHING©: BLOW & LIFT

REQUIRED MATERIALS

- ☑ PULSE OXIMETER
- ☑ SUPPLEMENTAL OXYGEN, IF PRESCRIBED
- ☑ CHAIR WITH NO ARMS
- ☑ WATER (GLASS OR BOTTLE)

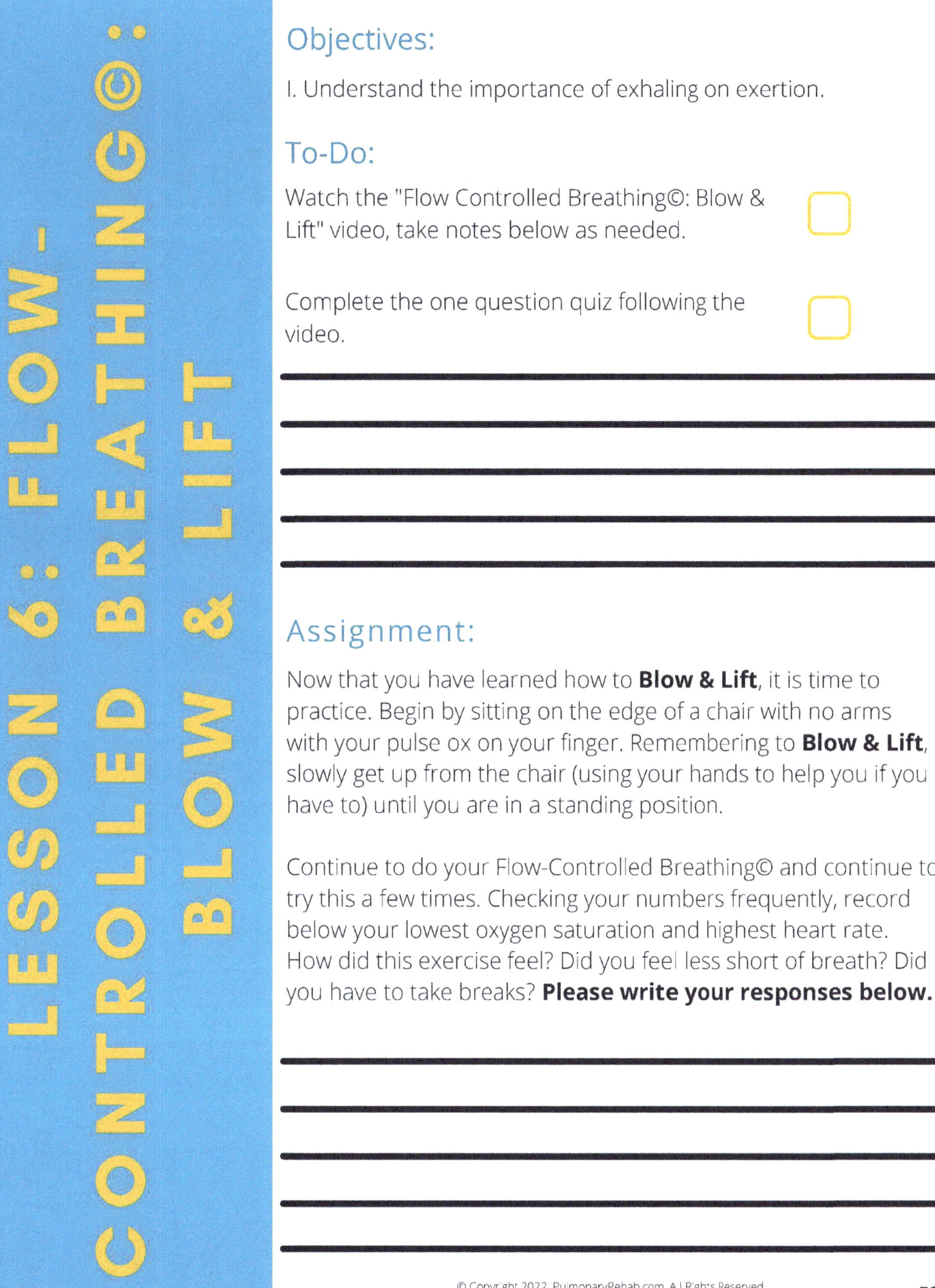

LESSON 6: FLOW-CONTROLLED BREATHING©: BLOW & LIFT

Objectives:

I. Understand the importance of exhaling on exertion.

To-Do:

- [ ] Watch the "Flow Controlled Breathing©: Blow & Lift" video, take notes below as needed.
- [ ] Complete the one question quiz following the video.

Assignment:

Now that you have learned how to **Blow & Lift**, it is time to practice. Begin by sitting on the edge of a chair with no arms with your pulse ox on your finger. Remembering to **Blow & Lift**, slowly get up from the chair (using your hands to help you if you have to) until you are in a standing position.

Continue to do your Flow-Controlled Breathing© and continue to try this a few times. Checking your numbers frequently, record below your lowest oxygen saturation and highest heart rate. How did this exercise feel? Did you feel less short of breath? Did you have to take breaks? **Please write your responses below.**

LESSON 7: CLIMBING STAIRS WITH FLOW-CONTROLLED BREATHING©

REQUIRED MATERIALS

- ☑ PULSE OXIMETER
- ☑ SUPPLEMENTAL OXYGEN, IF PRESCRIBED
- ☑ STAIRS
- ☑ WATER (GLASS OR BOTTLE)

LESSON 7: INTRODUCTION TO THE STAIR CLIMBING LOG

Objectives:

I. Understand the importance of the **Stair Climbing Log** and how to use it in this course.

II. Use the **Stair Climbing Log** to capture the number of steps climbed, steps per exhalation, recovery time at the top of the stairs, oxygen saturation, and heart rate during stair climbing.

To-Do:

Watch the "Introduction to the Stair Climbing Log" video, take notes below as needed. ☐

Assignment:

Continue on to watch the instructional video on how to incorporate Flow-Controlled Breathing© with climbing stairs.

When you're ready to practice, use the **Stair Climbing Log** on the next page to record your numbers and **write any observations below.**

LESSON 7: INTRODUCTION TO THE STAIR CLIMBING LOG

Use the log below to record the number of steps, steps per exhalation. number of rests, recovery time at top of stairs, pre/during/post oxygen saturation and heart rate, and amount of supplemental oxygen used if applicable. If you capture multiple oxygen saturation and heart rate values during exercise, please record the lowest oxygen saturation and highest heart rate. If needed, please refer to the "Introduction to the Stair Climbing Log" located in this lesson for a refresher on what this form is and how to use it.

Please circle any oxygen saturation below 92%.

Date	Number of Steps	Steps per Exhalation	Number of Rests	Recovery Time at Top of Stairs (min)	Oxygen Saturation (%)	Heart Rate (bpm)	Oxygen (L) or Room Air
					Pre: During: After:	Pre: During: After:	Pre: During: After:
					Pre: During: After:	Pre: During: After:	Pre: During: After:
					Pre: During: After:	Pre: During: After:	Pre: During: After:
					Pre: During: After:	Pre: During: After:	Pre: During: After:

LESSON 7: CLIMBING STAIRS WITH FLOW-CONTROLLED BREATHING©

Objectives:

I. Understand how to combine Flow-Controlled Breathing© with stair climbing.

II. Understand that it is critical to only climb up the stairs when you are exhaling.

III. Understand the importance of allowing your breathing to dictate the pace at which you climb the stairs, NOT the other way around.

IV. Understand the steps you should take should you get winded while going up the stairs, including once you reach the top of the stairs.

V. Use the **Shortness of Breath Scale** to quantify your shortness of breath after completing Climbing Stairs with Flow-Controlled Breathing©.

VI. Use the **Work Scale** to quantify the amount of work being done during "Climbing Stairs with Flow-Controlled Breathing©".

To-Do:

- [ ] Watch the "Climbing Stairs with Flow Controlled Breathing©" video, take notes below as needed.
- [ ] Complete the one question quiz following the video.

LESSON 7: CLIMBING STAIRS WITH FLOW-CONTROLLED BREATHING©

Assignment:

Now that you have learned how to incorporate Flow-Controlled Breathing© with stair-climbing, it is time to practice. Record any observations on page 55. Then use the **Stair-Climbing Log** located on **page 56**, to record your numbers.

To-Do:

After completing Climbing Stairs with Flow-Controlled Breathing©, use the **Shortness of Breath Scale** below to quantify your shortness of breath by circling the column containing the shortness of breath number that best describes how you feel.

***If you need a refresher on what this scale is and how to use it, please reference the video in Section 2 Lesson 4 entitled "Introduction to the Shortness of Breath Scale".*

Shortness of Breath Scale

SOB #	0	½	1	2	3	4	5	6	7	8
SEVERITY	NONE	JUST NOTICEABLE	VERY SLIGHT	SLIGHT	MODERATE	MORE MODERATE	SEVERE	MORE SEVERE	VERY SEVERE	MAXIMUM
	Normal Speech				Choppy Speech		Can't Speak		Call 911!	

LESSON 7: CLIMBING STAIRS WITH FLOW-CONTROLLED BREATHING©

To-Do:

After completing Climbing Stairs with Flow-Controlled Breathing© , use the **Work Scale** below to quantify the amount of work you performed completing these exercises by circling the column containing the work number that best describes how you feel.

You may designate a number for each exercise or choose a number that best represents the amount of work performed throughout the entire menu.

***If you need a refresher on what this scale is and how to use it, please reference the video in Section 3 Lesson 4 entitled "Introduction to the Work Scale".*

How difficult is the exercise that you are doing right now?

This is no work at all	Not bad at all, but too easy	A little harder, but still good	This is good, I'm challenged	Getting too difficult	Nope, can't do it
0	1	2	3	4	5

LESSON 7: CLIMBING STAIRS WITH FLOW-CONTROLLED BREATHING©

Assignment:

Take a few minutes and reflect on the number you chose from the **Shortness of Breath Scale**.

- Was it what you expected?
- Was it higher or lower than you expected?

Using Flow-Controlled Breathing©, did you notice less shortness of breath climbing the stairs as well as when you got to the top, compared to when you usually climb stairs?

If you know what your oxygen saturation is when you usually climb stairs, please write it down below and compare it to the oxygen saturation numbers you captured in the **Stair Climbing Log**. Reflect on the differences between them.

Hopefully, you noticed a decrease in your shortness of breath and an increase in your oxygen saturation compared to when you usually climb stairs. If you did not, please continue to practice incorporating the Flow-Controlled Breathing© technique with climbing stairs until you notice an improvement in your shortness of breath as well as your oxygen saturation.

If you did have a noticeable improvement in your shortness of breath, **congratulations**! Keep up the good work!

Record any other notable observations below.

Assignment:

Take a few minutes and reflect on the number you chose from the Work Scale.

- Was it what you expected?
- Was it higher or lower than you expected?
- If it was not in the **ideal 2-3.5 range**, what do you plan to do differently next time?
- Using Flow-Controlled Breathing©, did you feel as though you were performing less work to climb the stairs compared to when you usually climb stairs?

If the number was above this **2-3.5 range**, by continuing to exercise your muscles will strengthen and you will see a noticeable decrease in the amount of work required to do this same activity.

If you did have a noticeable decrease in the amount of work required, **congratulations**! Keep up the good work! Continue to practice this method every time you climb the stairs.

Record any other notable observations below.

Section 4

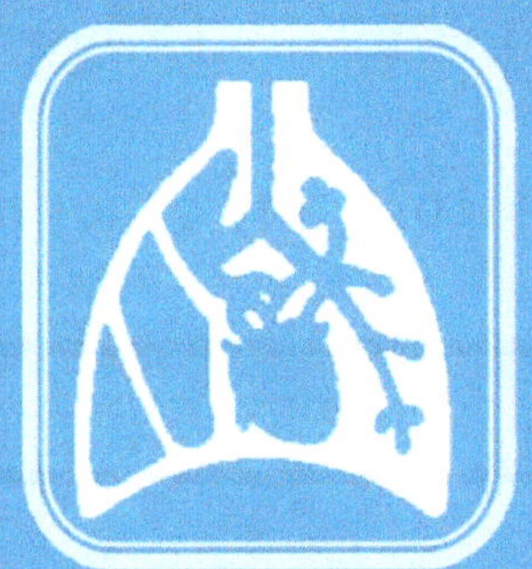

THOUGHT OF THE DAY...

HAVING A ROUGH DAY?

PLACE YOUR HAND OVER YOUR HEART.

FEEL THAT?

THAT'S CALLED *purpose.*

YOU'RE ALIVE FOR A REASON.

DON'T GIVE UP.

LESSON 1: CONGRATULATIONS!

To-Do:

Watch "Congratulations" video. 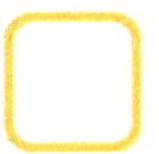

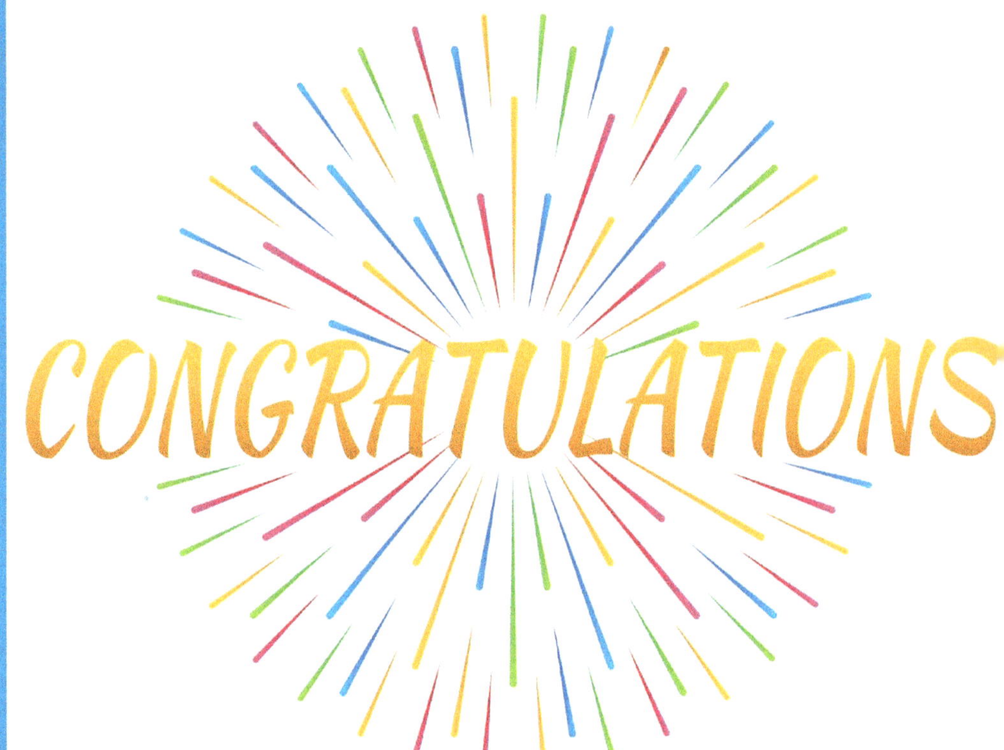

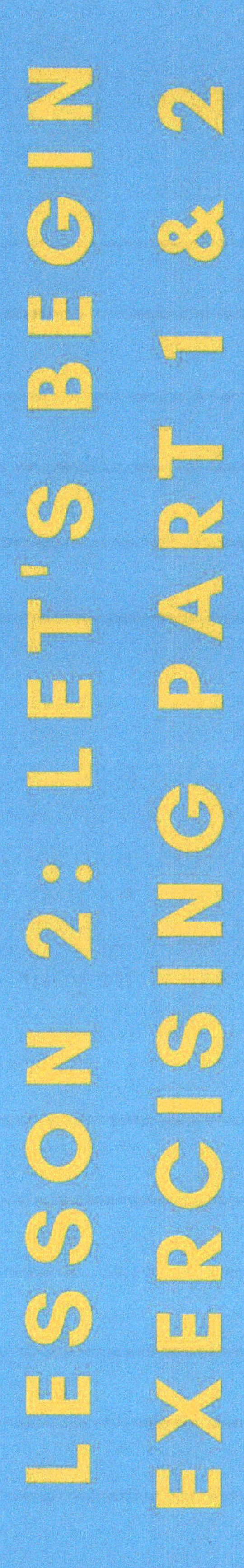

Objectives:

I. Be able to define and describe what a menu is and its various components.

II. Understand how to incorporate posture with the exercises.

III. Understand common compensations of exercises in this course.

IV. Understand how to use a pulse oximeter to get accurate readings of your oxygen saturation and heart rate during exercise.

V. Understand the importance of filling out the **Pulse Oximeter Log** in this course.

To-Do:

Watch the "Let's Begin Exercising! (Part 1)" video, take notes below as needed. ☐

LESSON 1: LET'S BEGIN EXERCISING PART 1 & 2

To-Do:

Watch the "Let's Begin Exercising! (Part 2)" video, take notes below as needed.

Assignment:

Before moving on to the exercise component of the course, please take a few minutes to reflect on how you feel about exercise--is it something that makes you anxious or stressed, do you see it as a stress reliever? When was the last time that you exercised? What are some goals you have for yourself going into the exercise component of the course? **Please write your responses below.**

LESSON 3: BEFORE WE BEGIN... LET'S GET OUR MATERIALS

REQUIRED MATERIALS

- ☑ PULSE OXIMETER
- ☑ SUPPLEMENTAL OXYGEN, IF PRESCRIBED
- ☑ 2-5 LB WEIGHTS OR AT-HOME SUBSTITUTIONS
- ☑ STRAIGHT WALL
- ☑ ITEM FOR BACK SUPPORT (I.E. PILLOW, YOGA MAT)
- ☑ ITEM FOR SUPPORT (I.E. KITCHEN COUNTER, LOCKED ROLLING WALKER)
- ☑ CHAIR WITH NO ARMS
- ☑ TIMER
- ☑ TOWEL ROLL
- ☑ KNEE STRAP OR BELT
- ☑ WATER (GLASS OR BOTTLE)
- ☑ TREADMILL (IF APPLICABLE)

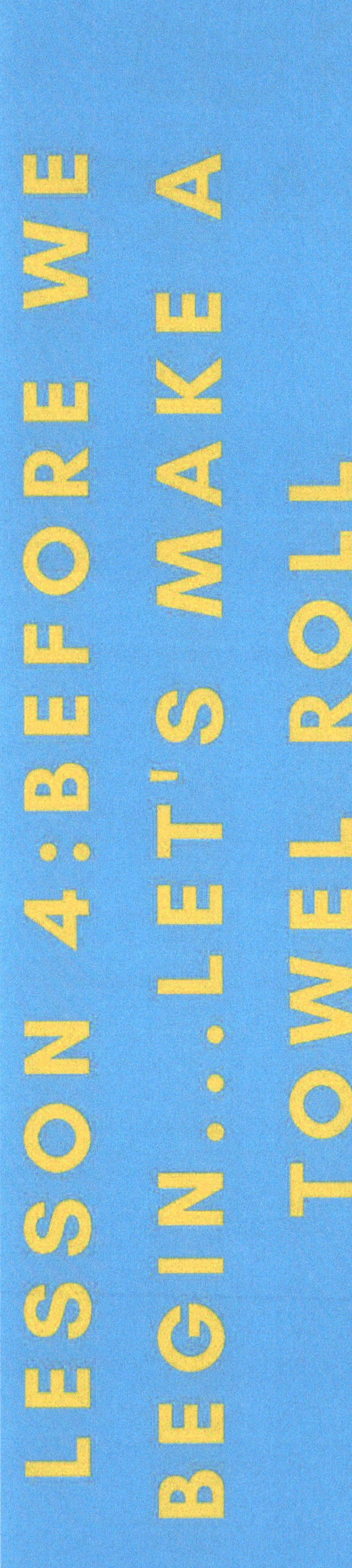
LESSON 4:BEFORE WE
BEGIN..LET'S MAKE A
TOWEL ROLL

Objectives:

I. Understand how to make a towel roll.

II. Successfully make your own towel roll to be used during specific exercises throughout the rest of the course.

To-Do:

Watch the "Let's Make a Towel Roll" video, take notes below as needed.

Assignment:

Now it's time to make your own towel roll! Please use the instructional video as your guide and follow along.

This towel roll is very important as it is required for some of the exercises contained in the subsequent menus in this section of the course. Once you successfully make your towel roll you're ready to move on to the next lesson where your first exercise menu will be introduced.

LESSON 5: SUKI'S SEATED POWER MENU

Objectives:

I. To stretch and strengthen lower body muscle groups while seated, thus reducing workload on your weight bearing joints, lungs, and heart.

II. Use the **Shortness of Breath Scale** to quantify your shortness of breath after completing **Suki's Seated Power Menu**.

III. Use the **Work Scale** to quantify the amount of work being done during **Suki's Seated Power Menu**.

To-Do:

Watch the "What is Suki's Seated Power Menu" video, take notes below as needed. ☐

LESSON 5: SUKI'S SEATED POWER MENU

REQUIRED MATERIALS

- ☑ PULSE OXIMETER
- ☑ SUPPLEMENTAL OXYGEN, IF PRESCRIBED
- ☑ CHAIR WITH NO ARMS
- ☑ TOWEL ROLL
- ☑ KNEE STRAP OR BELT
- ☑ WATER (GLASS OR BOTTLE)

LESSON 5: SUKI'S SEATED POWER MENU

To-Do:

Look at chart of exercises, including sets and set/time. Familiarize yourself with exercise names. ☐

Watch the "Menu #1: Suki's Seated Power Menu" video, take notes below as needed. ☐

Important Reminders:

1) Proper posture (squared feet, pinched shoulders, level chin, no leaning)

2) Blow & Lift while doing Flow-Controlled Breathing©

3) Go slowly

4) Stop when winded

5) Have fun! You're **not** just exercising, *you're working towards your goal!*

Assignment:

Now it is time to begin practicing this menu. Feel free to have the exercise video playing to help guide you. Use **Self-Assessment #4** beginning on **page 76** to record your numbers and answer the corresponding questions.

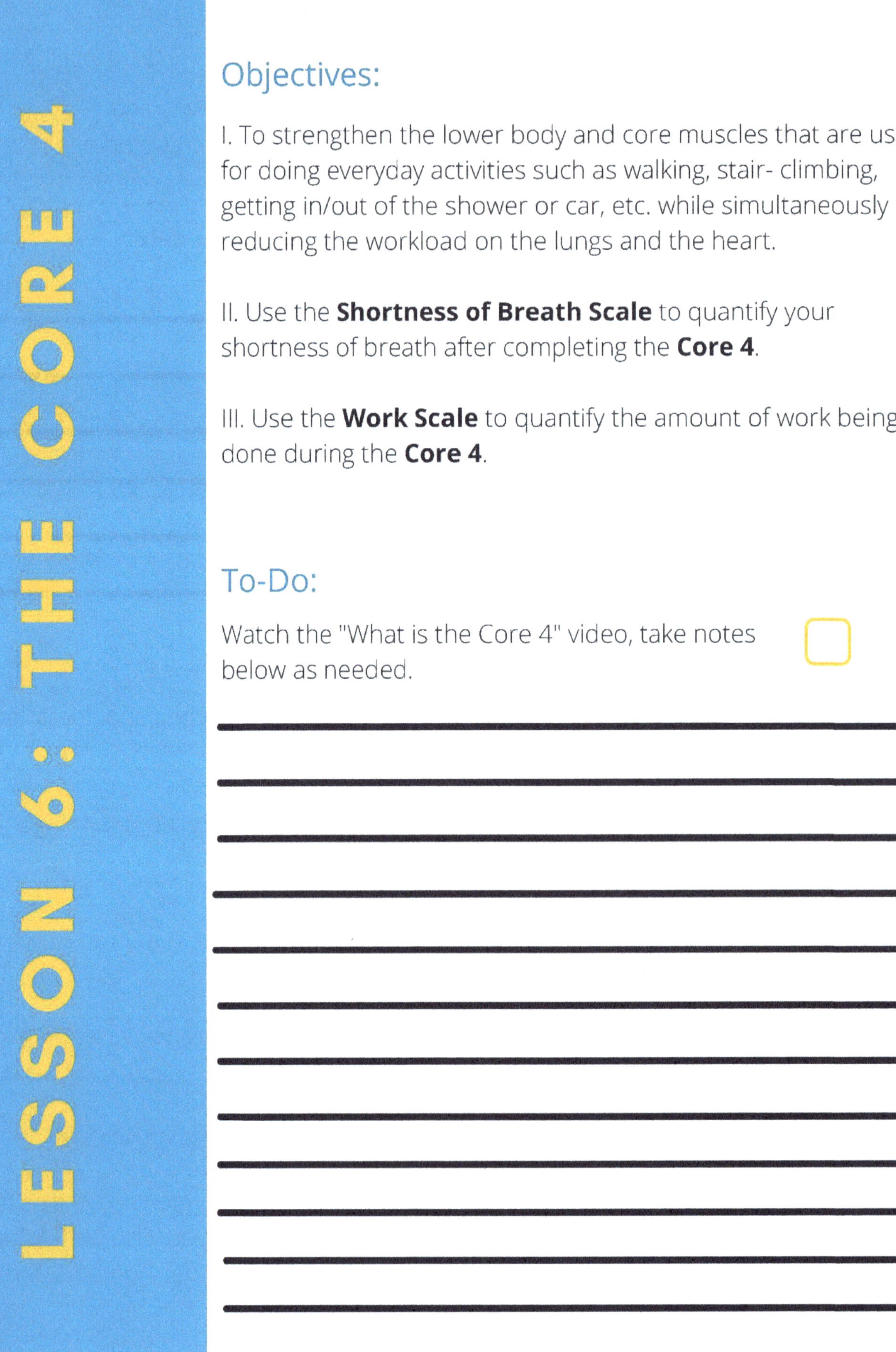

LESSON 6: THE CORE 4

Objectives:

I. To strengthen the lower body and core muscles that are used for doing everyday activities such as walking, stair- climbing, getting in/out of the shower or car, etc. while simultaneously reducing the workload on the lungs and the heart.

II. Use the **Shortness of Breath Scale** to quantify your shortness of breath after completing the **Core 4**.

III. Use the **Work Scale** to quantify the amount of work being done during the **Core 4**.

To-Do:

Watch the "What is the Core 4" video, take notes below as needed. ☐

REQUIRED MATERIALS

- ☑ PULSE OXIMETER
- ☑ SUPPLEMENTAL OXYGEN, IF PRESCRIBED
- ☑ ITEM FOR SUPPORT (I.E. KITCHEN COUNTER, LOCKED ROLLING WALKER)
- ☑ CHAIR WITH NO ARMS
- ☑ WATER (GLASS OR BOTTLE)

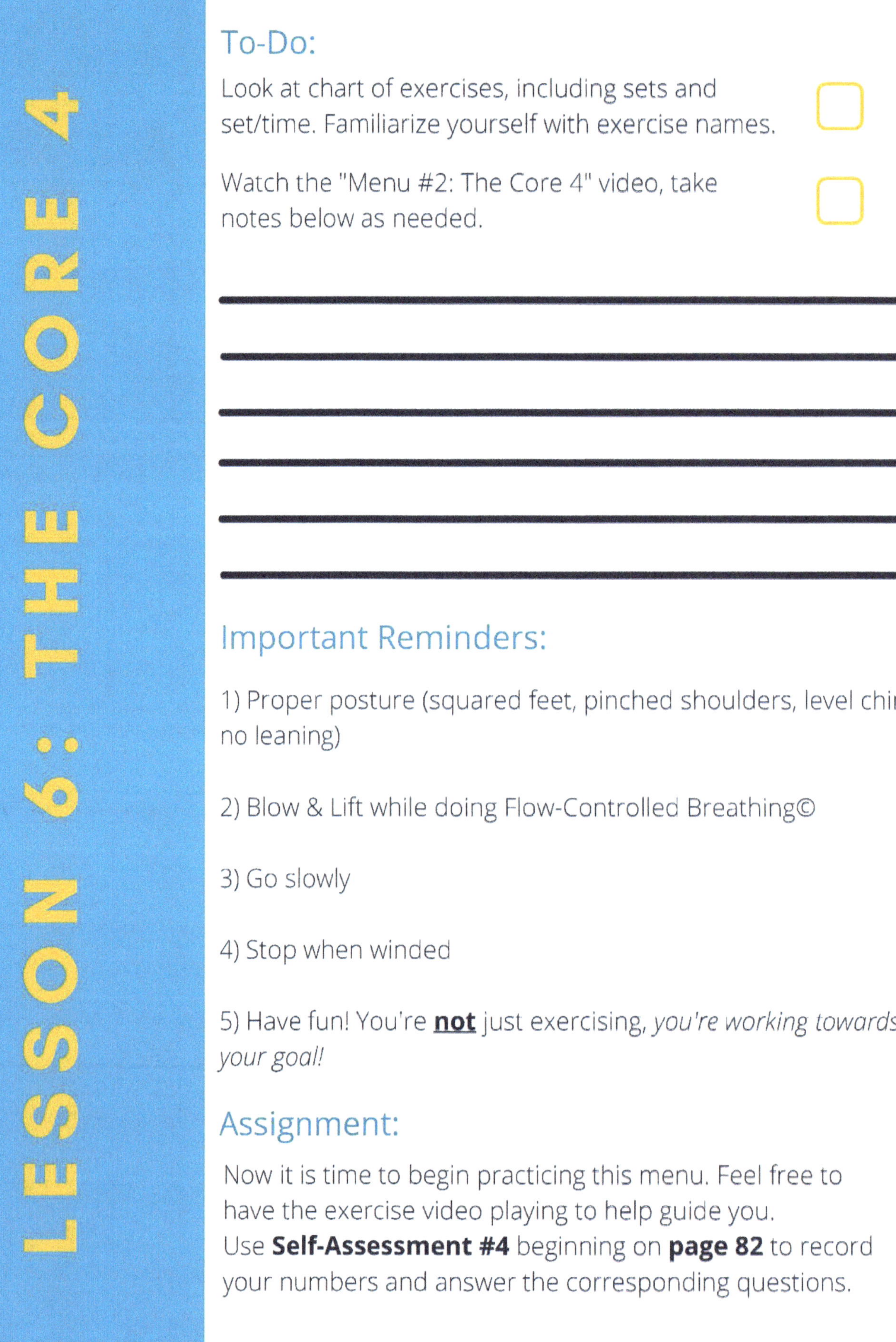

LESSON 6: THE CORE 4

To-Do:

- [ ] Look at chart of exercises, including sets and set/time. Familiarize yourself with exercise names.
- [ ] Watch the "Menu #2: The Core 4" video, take notes below as needed.

Important Reminders:

1) Proper posture (squared feet, pinched shoulders, level chin, no leaning)

2) Blow & Lift while doing Flow-Controlled Breathing©

3) Go slowly

4) Stop when winded

5) Have fun! You're **not** just exercising, *you're working towards your goal!*

Assignment:

Now it is time to begin practicing this menu. Feel free to have the exercise video playing to help guide you.
Use **Self-Assessment #4** beginning on **page 82** to record your numbers and answer the corresponding questions.

LESSON 7: INTRODUCTION TO SELF-ASSESMENT #4

Objectives:

I. Understand the purpose and contents of **Self-Assessment #4**.

II. Understand how to use **Self-Assessment #4**.

To-Do:

Watch the "Introduction to Self-Assessment #4" video, take notes below as needed. ☐

Assignment:

Before continuing on to complete **Self-Assessment #4**, please take some time to continue to familiarize yourself with **Self-Assessment #4** by flipping through the next 14 pages in this workbook. Take notes below as needed.

LESSON 7: SELF-ASSESSMENT #4

CAPTURING AND RECORDING YOUR INITIAL NUMBERS: SUKI'S SEATED POWER MENU & THE CORE 4

Objectives:

I. Reflect on **Suki's Seated Power Menu** and **Core 4** and to quantitatively compare your oxygen saturation and heart rate during various exercises in these menus.

II. Establish a reference point when comparing oxygen saturation and heart rate at this point in the program in comparison to other checkpoints in the program to quantify your progress.

III. Allows for quantification of shortness of breath after **Suki's Seated Power Menu** and the **Core 4** using the **Shortness of Breath Scale**.

IV. Provides a quantitative comparison of shortness of breath after **Suki's Seated Power Menu** vs. the **Core 4** using the **Shortness of Breath Scale**.

V. Allows for a quantification of the amount of work being performed after **Suki's Seated Power Menu** vs. the **Core 4** using the **Work Scale**.

VI. Provides a quantitative comparison of the amount of work being performed after **Suki's Seated Power Menu** vs. the **Core 4** using the **Work Scale**.

LESSON 7: SELF-ASSESSMENT #4

CAPTURING AND RECORDING YOUR INITIAL NUMBERS: SUKI'S SEATED POWER MENU & THE CORE 4

To-Do:

After watching the explanation of **Suki's Seated Power Menu** and familiarizing yourself with the exercises by looking at the chart as well as watching the step-by-step exercise guide for this menu, begin doing the exercises in the order they appear both in the aforementioned chart and video.

Be sure to take rests when you are feeling short of breath as well as between each exercise as needed. Check and record your oxygen saturation and heart rate using your pulse oximeter both before, during, and after exercising. Please record these numbers in the tables on the next page.

As a reminder, put the pulse oximeter on your finger and wait about 20 seconds to allow the device to capture the most accurate readings. If you find that your oxygen saturation and heart rate readings are much different than your normal readings, please put the device on your other hand, trying multiple fingers until you get the best signal strength and reading.

Try your best to capture 2-3 oxygen saturation and heart rate readings from your pulse oximeter ***DURING*** the time you are walking and separate each below in the appropriate box with commas. Lastly but certainly not least, **remember to do your Flow-Controlled Breathing©**!

As a reminder, please check your oxygen saturation and heart rate readings frequently during this exercise. If you find that your oxygen saturation drops below or your heart rate goes above the accepted values your healthcare providers gave to you, immediately stop.

Reminder: I usually recommend maintaining an oxygen saturation of 92% or higher.

LESSON 7:
SELF-ASSESSMENT #4

CAPTURING AND RECORDING YOUR INITIAL NUMBERS: SUKI'S SEATED POWER MENU & THE CORE 4

Pulse Oximeter Reading (Before exercise)

Oxygen Saturation (%)	
Heart Rate (bpm)	
Supplemental Oxygen (L) *(if you don't wear oxygen, write "room air")*	

Pulse Oximeter Reading
(During exercise; multiple readings separated by commas)

Oxygen Saturation (%)	
Heart Rate (bpm)	
Supplemental Oxygen (L) *(if you don't wear oxygen, write "room air")*	
Number of rests	

Pulse Oximeter Reading (After exercise)

Oxygen Saturation (%)	
Heart Rate (bpm)	
Supplemental Oxygen (L) *(if you don't wear oxygen, write "room air")*	

LESSON 7: SELF-ASSESSMENT #4

CAPTURING AND RECORDING YOUR INITIAL NUMBERS: SUKI'S SEATED POWER MENU & THE CORE 4

Reflection:

- How did that menu make you feel--were you short of breath? If you were short of breath, were you doing your Flow-Controlled Breathing© or possibly going through the exercises too fast?
- What muscles did you feel working?
- Was it challenging?
- Were some exercises harder than others and if so, which ones?
- How did your oxygen saturation and heart rate compare before, during, and after exercise?
- What has improved? Can you feel these improvements?
- When you go to do this menu again in the future what are some of your goals?

Please record your responses to the above questions in the space below.

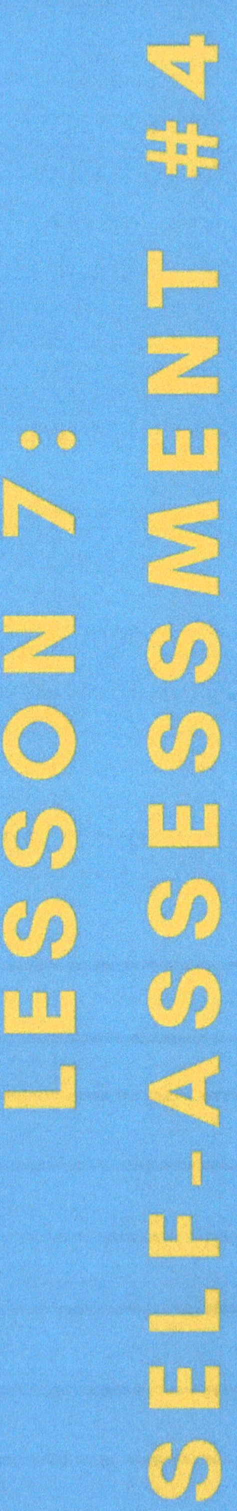

CAPTURING AND RECORDING YOUR INITIAL NUMBERS: SUKI'S SEATED POWER MENU & THE CORE 4

After completing **Suki's Seated Power Menu**, use the **Shortness of Breath Scale** below to quantify your shortness of breath by circling the column containing the shortness of breath number that best describes how you feel.

***If you need a refresher on what this scale is and how to use it, please reference the video in Section 2 Lesson 4 entitled "Introduction to the Shortness of Breath Scale".*

Shortness of Breath Scale

SOB #	0	½	1	2	3	4	5	6	7	8
SEVERITY	NONE	JUST NOTICEABLE	VERY SLIGHT	SLIGHT	MODERATE	MORE MODERATE	SEVERE	MORE SEVERE	VERY SEVERE	MAXIMUM
	Normal Speech				Choppy Speech		Can't Speak		Call 911!	

LESSON 7: SELF-ASSESSMENT #4

CAPTURING AND RECORDING YOUR INITIAL NUMBERS: SUKI'S SEATED POWER MENU & THE CORE 4

After completing **Suki's Seated Power Menu**, use the **Work Scale** below to quantify the amount of work you performed completing these exercises by circling the column containing the work number that best describes how you feel.

You may designate a number for each exercise or choose a number that best represents the amount of work performed throughout the entire menu.

***If you need a refresher on what this scale is and how to use it, please reference the video in Section 3 Lesson 4 entitled "Introduction to the Work Scale".*

How difficult is the exercise that you are doing right now?

This is no work at all	Not bad at all, but too easy	A little harder, but still good	This is good, I'm challenged	Getting too difficult	Nope, can't do it
0	1	2	3	4	5

Let's try and stay between 2 and 3.5

LESSON 7:
SELF-ASSESSMENT #4

CAPTURING AND RECORDING YOUR INITIAL NUMBERS: SUKI'S SEATED POWER MENU & THE CORE 4

To-Do:

After watching the explanation of the **Core 4** and familiarizing yourself with the exercises by looking at the chart as well as watching the step-by-step exercise guide for this menu, begin doing the exercises in the order they appear both in the aforementioned chart and video.

Be sure to take rests when you are feeling short of breath as well as between each exercise as needed. Check and record your oxygen saturation and heart rate using your pulse oximeter both before, during, and after exercising. Please record these numbers in the tables on the next page.

As a reminder, put the pulse oximeter on your finger and wait about 20 seconds to allow the device to capture the most accurate readings. If you find that your oxygen saturation and heart rate readings are much different than your normal readings, please put the device on your other hand, trying multiple fingers until you get the best signal strength and reading.

Try your best to capture 2-3 oxygen saturation and heart rate readings from your pulse oximeter ***DURING*** the time you are walking and separate each below in the appropriate box with commas. Lastly but certainly not least, **remember to do your Flow-Controlled Breathing©!**

As a reminder, please check your oxygen saturation and heart rate readings frequently during this exercise and if you find that your oxygen saturation drops below **(usually 92%)** or your heart rate goes above the accepted values your healthcare providers gave to you, immediately stop.

LESSON 7:
SELF-ASSESSMENT #4

CAPTURING AND RECORDING YOUR INITIAL NUMBERS: SUKI'S SEATED POWER MENU & THE CORE 4

Pulse Oximeter Reading (Before exercise)

Oxygen Saturation (%)	
Heart Rate (bpm)	
Supplemental Oxygen (L) *(if you don't wear oxygen, write "room air")*	

Pulse Oximeter Reading
(During exercise; multiple readings separated by commas)

Oxygen Saturation (%)	
Heart Rate (bpm)	
Supplemental Oxygen (L) *(if you don't wear oxygen, write "room air")*	
Number of rests	

Pulse Oximeter Reading (After exercise)

Oxygen Saturation (%)	
Heart Rate (bpm)	
Supplemental Oxygen (L) *(if you don't wear oxygen, write "room air")*	

LESSON 7: SELF-ASSESSMENT #4

CAPTURING AND RECORDING YOUR INITIAL NUMBERS: SUKI'S SEATED POWER MENU & THE CORE 4

Reflection:

- How did that menu make you feel--were you short of breath? If you were short of breath, were you doing Flow-Controlled Breathing© or possibly going through the exercises too fast?
- What muscles did you feel working?
- Was it challenging?
- Were some exercises harder than others and if so which ones?
- How did your oxygen saturation and heart rate compare before, during, and after exercise?
- What has improved? Can you feel these improvements?
- When you go to do this menu again in the future what are some of your goals?

Please record your responses to the above questions in the space below.

LESSON 7: SELF-ASSESSMENT #4

CAPTURING AND RECORDING YOUR INITIAL NUMBERS: SUKI'S SEATED POWER MENU & THE CORE 4

After completing the **Core 4**, use the **Shortness of Breath Scale** below to quantify your shortness of breath by circling the column containing the shortness of breath number that best describes how you feel.

***If you need a refresher on what this scale is and how to use it, please reference the video in Section 2 Lesson 4 entitled "Introduction to the Shortness of Breath Scale".*

Shortness of Breath Scale

SOB #	0	½	1	2	3	4	5	6	7	8
SEVERITY	NONE	JUST NOTICEABLE	VERY SLIGHT	SLIGHT	MODERATE	MORE MODERATE	SEVERE	MORE SEVERE	VERY SEVERE	MAXIMUM
	Normal Speech				Choppy Speech		Can't Speak		Call 911!	

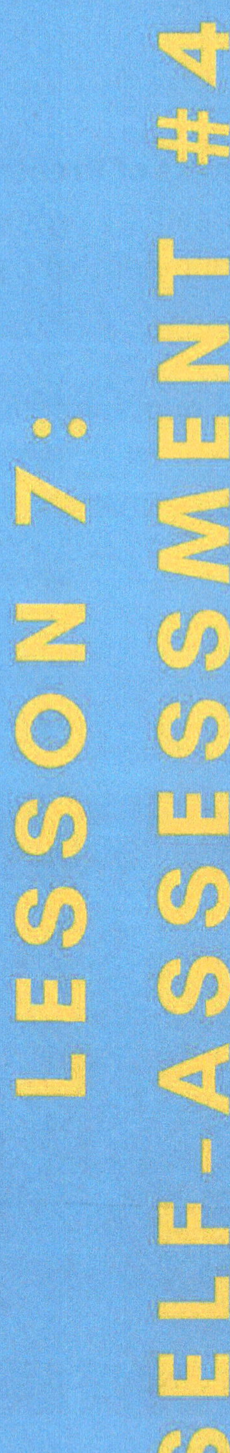

CAPTURING AND RECORDING YOUR INITIAL NUMBERS: SUKI'S SEATED POWER MENU & THE CORE 4

Reflection:

Take a few minutes and compare the shortness of breath numbe you chose after **Suki's Seated Power Menu (page 80)** versus the one you chose after the **Core 4 (page 85).** Which number is higher? Does the higher number reflect the menu that you felt was more difficult?

We ideally want you to be breathing at a 2-3 on this **Shortness of Breath Scale**, did you remain within this range during both exercises menus? If not, reflect on why your shortness of breath selection may have been above or below this range (i.e. consider your pace and your proper use of the Flow-Controlled Breathing© technique).

Also, please keep in mind that your shortness of breath selection for these menus may differ as one menu is done sitting while the other is done standing. As you continue to progress through this course you will get stronger and have decreased shortness of breath, allowing you to successfully complete exercises that you were not able to do before. Keep up the good work!

Please record your responses to the above questions in the space below.

LESSON 7: SELF-ASSESSMENT #4

CAPTURING AND RECORDING YOUR INITIAL NUMBERS: SUKI'S SEATED POWER MENU & THE CORE 4

After completing the **Core 4**, use the **Work Scale** below to quantify the amount of work you performed completing these exercises by circling the column containing the work number that best describes how you feel. You may designate a number for each exercise or choose a number that best represents the amount of work performed throughout the entire menu.

***If you need a refresher on what this scale is and how to use it, please reference the video in Section 3 Lesson 4 entitled "Introduction to the Work Scale".*

How difficult is the exercise that you are doing right now?

This is no work at all	Not bad at all, but too easy	A little harder, but still good	This is good, I'm challenged	Getting too difficult	Nope, can't do it
0	1	2	3	4	5

<u>Let's try and stay between 2 and 3.5</u>

LESSON 7: SELF-ASSESSMENT #4

CAPTURING AND RECORDING YOUR INITIAL NUMBERS: SUKI'S SEATED POWER MENU & THE CORE 4

Reflection:

Take a few minutes and compare the work number you chose after **Suki's Seated Power Menu (page 81)** versus the one you chose after the **Core 4 (page 87)**.

- Which number is higher?
- Does the higher number reflect the menu that you felt was more difficult?

We ideally want you to be breathing at a **2-3.5** on this **Work Scale**, did you remain within this range during both exercises menus? If not, reflect on why your work selection may have been above or below this range (i.e. going too slow and/or fast, not using the Flow-Controlled Breathing© technique, using too heavy of a weight, doing too many repetitions, etc.).

Also, please keep in mind that your **Work Scale** selections for these menus may differ as one menu is done sitting while the other is done standing. As you continue to progress through this course, you will get stronger and your **Work Scale** number will decrease, allowing you to successfully complete exercises that you were not able to do before. Keep up the good work!

Please record your responses to the above questions in the space below.

LESSON 7: SELF-ASSESSMENT #4

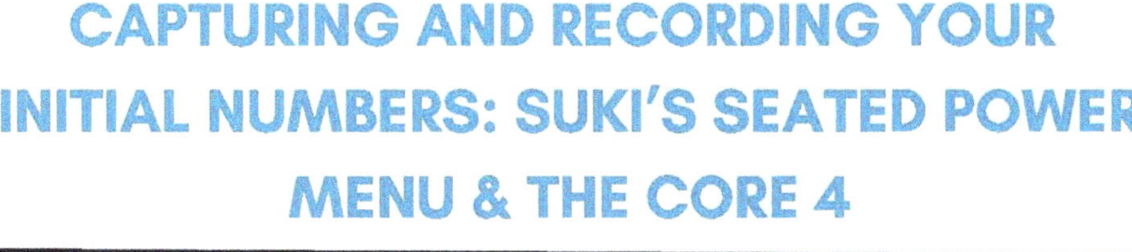

CAPTURING AND RECORDING YOUR INITIAL NUMBERS: SUKI'S SEATED POWER MENU & THE CORE 4

Reflection:

Using the space below, take a few minutes to reflect on your experience doing **Suki's Seated Power Menu** and the **Core 4**.

- Was one menu more difficult than the other?
- How was your balance?
- Compare your oxygen saturation and heart rate before, during, and after for **Suki's Seated Power Menu** and the **Core 4**. What has improved? Can you feel these improvements?
- Write down any goals you have for yourself after completing these menus.

If you did have trouble with either of these menus, it is okay - as you progress through this program, you will get stronger, your balance will improve, and overall these exercises will become easier!

Great job, you've completed your fourth assessment! Make sure that all the information is filled out and keep this assessment in a safe place.

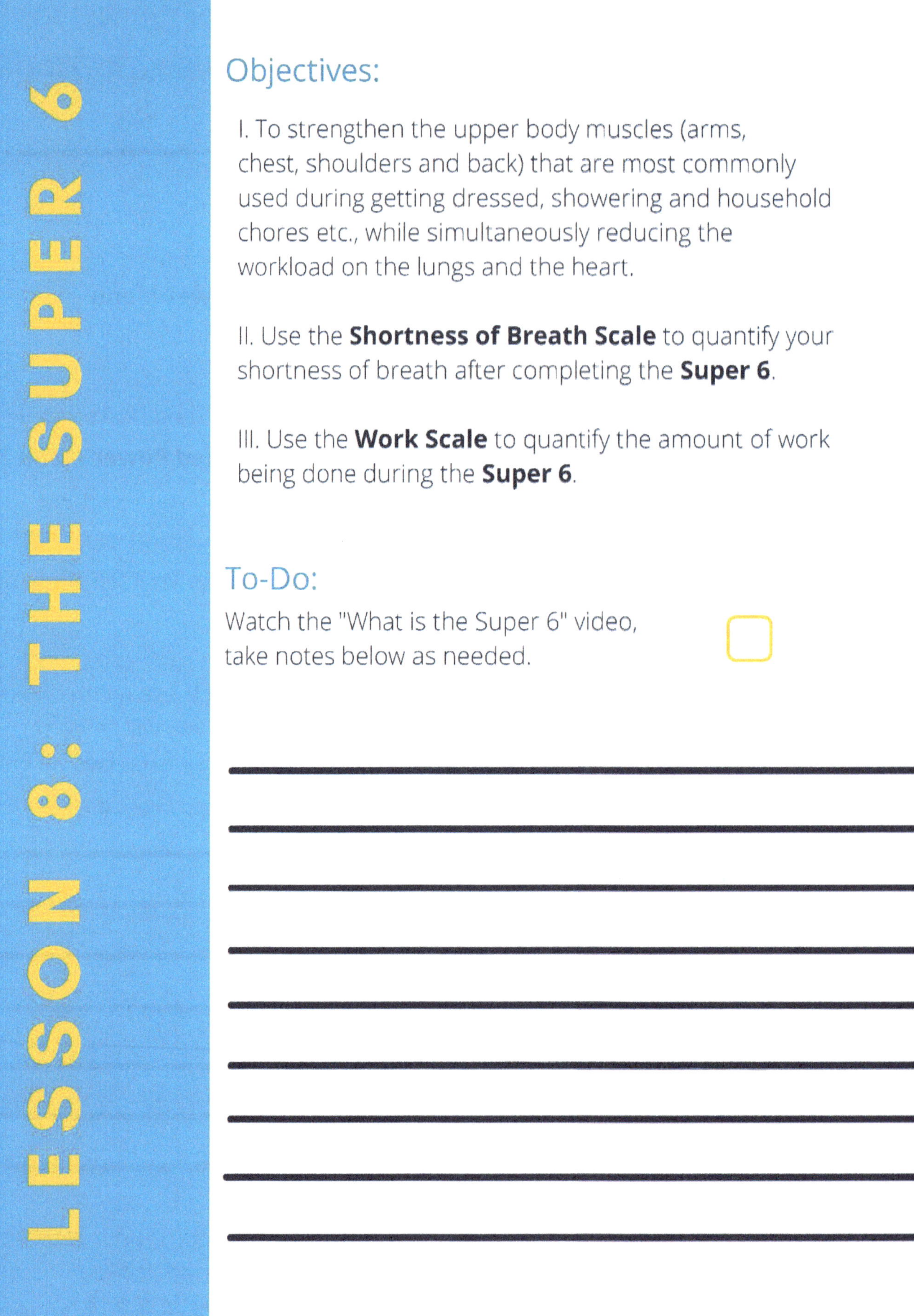

Objectives:

I. To strengthen the upper body muscles (arms, chest, shoulders and back) that are most commonly used during getting dressed, showering and household chores etc., while simultaneously reducing the workload on the lungs and the heart.

II. Use the **Shortness of Breath Scale** to quantify your shortness of breath after completing the **Super 6**.

III. Use the **Work Scale** to quantify the amount of work being done during the **Super 6**.

To-Do:

Watch the "What is the Super 6" video, take notes below as needed. ☐

REQUIRED MATERIALS

- ☑ PULSE OXIMETER
- ☑ SUPPLEMENTAL OXYGEN, IF PRESCRIBED
- ☑ CHAIR WITH NO ARMS
- ☑ ITEM FOR BACK SUPPORT (I.E. PILLOW, YOGA MAT)
- ☑ 2-5 LB WEIGHTS OR AT-HOME SUBSTITUTIONS
- ☑ WATER (GLASS OR BOTTLE)

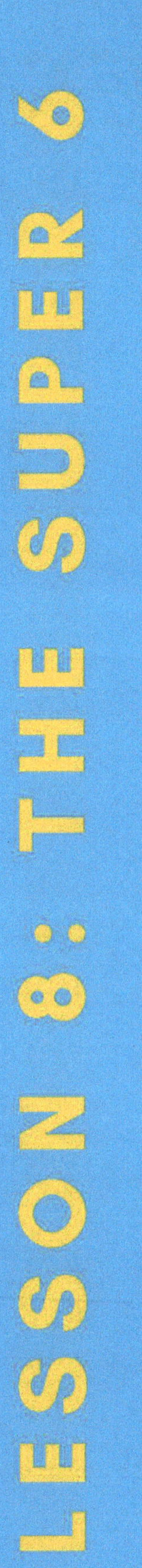

To-Do:

Look at chart of exercises, including sets and set/time. Familiarize yourself with exercise names. ☐

Watch the "Menu #2: The Super 6" video, take notes below as needed. ☐

Important Reminders:

1) Proper posture [squared feet, pinched shoulders, level chin, no leaning]

2) Blow & Lift while doing Flow-Controlled Breathing©

3) Go slowly

4) Stop when winded

5) Have fun! You're **not** just exercising, *you're working towards your goal!*

Assignment:

Now it is time to begin practicing this menu. Feel free to have the exercise video playing to help guide you. Use **Self-Assessment #5** beginning on **page 97** to record your numbers and answer the corresponding questions.

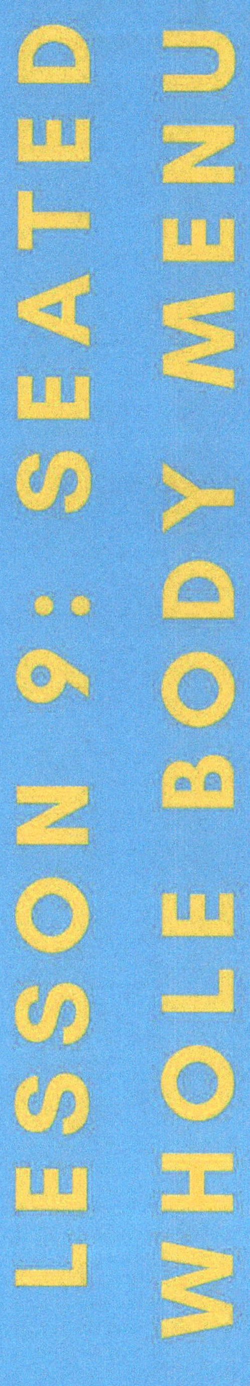

Objectives:

I. Stretch and tremendously strengthen the upper and lower body simultaneously while in a sitting position thus reducing the aerobic demand.

II. Use the **Shortness of Breath Scale** to quantify our shortness of breath after completing the **Seated Whole Body Menu.**

III. Use the **Work Scale** to quantify the amount of work being done during the **Seated Whole Body Menu.**

To-Do:

Watch the "What is the Seated Whole Body Menu" video, take notes below as needed. ☐

LESSON 9: SEATED WHOLE BODY MENU

REQUIRED MATERIALS

- ☑ PULSE OXIMETER
- ☑ SUPPLEMENTAL OXYGEN, IF PRESCRIBED
- ☑ CHAIR WITH NO ARMS
- ☑ ITEM FOR BACK SUPPORT (I.E. PILLOW, YOGA MAT)
- ☑ 2-5 LB WEIGHTS OR AT-HOME SUBSTITUTIONS
- ☑ TOWEL ROLL
- ☑ TIMER
- ☑ WATER (GLASS OR BOTTLE)

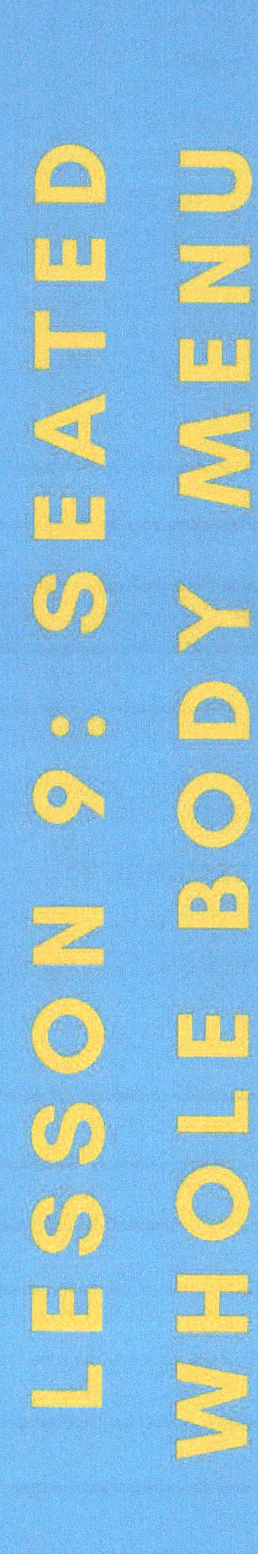

To-Do:

- [ ] Look at chart of exercises, including sets and set/time. Familiarize yourself with exercise names.
- [ ] Watch the "Menu #4: Seated Whole Body Menu" video, take notes below as needed.

Important Reminders:

1) Proper posture [squared feet, pinched shoulders, level chin, no leaning]

2) Blow & Lift while doing Flow-Controlled Breathing©

3) Go slowly

4) Stop when winded

5) Have fun! You're **<u>not</u>** just exercising, *you're working towards your goal!*

Assignment:

Now it is time to begin practicing this menu. Feel free to have the exercise video playing to help guide you. Use **Self-Assessment #5** beginning on **page 103** to record your numbers and answer the corresponding questions.

LESSON 10: INTRODUCTION TO SELF-ASSESSMENT #5

Objectives:

I. Understand the purpose and contents of **Self-Assessment #5**.

II. Understand how to use **Self-Assessment #5.**

To-Do:

Watch the "Introduction to Self-Assessment #5" video, take notes below as needed. ☐

Assignment:

Before continuing on to complete **Self-Assessment #5**, please take some time to continue to familiarize yourself with **Self-Assessment #5** by flipping through the next 14 pages in this workbook. Take notes below as needed.

LESSON 10:
SELF-ASSESSMENT #5

CAPTURING AND RECORDING YOUR INITIAL NUMBERS: THE SUPER 6 & SEATED WHOLE BODY MENU

Objectives:

I. Provides an opportunity to reflect on the **Super 6** and the **Seated Whole Body Menu** and to quantitatively compare your oxygen saturation and heart rate during various exercises in these menus.

II. Provides a reference point when comparing oxygen saturation and heart rate at this point in the program in comparison to other checkpoints in the program to quantify your progress.

III. Provides **quantification** of shortness of breath after the **Super 6** and the **Seated Whole Body Menu** using the **Shortness of Breath Scale**.

IV. Provides a **quantitative comparison** of shortness of breath after the **Super 6** and the **Seated Whole Body Menu** using the **Shortness of Breath Scale**.

V. Provides **quantification** of the amount of work being performed after the **Super 6** and the **Seated Whole Body Menu** using the **Work Scale**.

VI. Provides a **quantitative comparison** of the amount of work being performed after the **Super 6** and the **Seated Whole Body Menu** using the **Work Scale**.

LESSON 10:
SELF-ASSESSMENT #5

CAPTURING AND RECORDING YOUR INITIAL NUMBERS: THE SUPER 6 & SEATED WHOLE BODY MENU

To-Do:

After watching the explanation of the **Super 6** and familiarizing yourself with the exercises by looking at the chart as well as watching the step-by-step exercise guide for this menu, begin doing the exercises in the order they appear both in the aforementioned chart and video.

Be sure to take rests when you are feeling short of breath as well as between each exercise as needed. Check and record your oxygen saturation and heart rate using your pulse oximeter both before, during, and after exercising. Please record these numbers in the tables on the next page.

As a reminder, put the pulse ox on your finger and wait about 20 seconds to allow the device to capture the most accurate readings. If you find that your oxygen saturation and heart rate readings are much different than your normal readings, please put the device on your other hand, trying multiple fingers until you get the best signal strength and reading.

Try your best to capture 2-3 oxygen saturation and heart rate readings from your pulse oximeter ***DURING*** the time you are walking and separate each below in the appropriate box with commas. Lastly but certainly not least, **remember to do your Flow-Controlled Breathing©**!

As a reminder, please check your oxygen saturation and heart rate readings frequently during this exercise. If you find that your oxygen saturation drops below or your heart rate goes above the accepted values your healthcare providers gave to you, immediately stop.

Reminder: I usually recommend maintaining an oxygen saturation of 92% or higher.

LESSON 10:
SELF-ASSESSMENT #5

CAPTURING AND RECORDING YOUR INITIAL NUMBERS: THE SUPER 6 & SEATED WHOLE BODY MENU

Pulse Oximeter Reading (Before exercise)

Oxygen Saturation (%)	
Heart Rate (bpm)	
Supplemental Oxygen (L) *(if you don't wear oxygen, write "room air")*	

Pulse Oximeter Reading
(During exercise; multiple readings separated by commas)

Oxygen Saturation (%)	
Heart Rate (bpm)	
Supplemental Oxygen (L) *(if you don't wear oxygen, write "room air")*	
Number of rests	

Pulse Oximeter Reading (After exercise)

Oxygen Saturation (%)	
Heart Rate (bpm)	
Supplemental Oxygen (L) *(if you don't wear oxygen, write "room air")*	

LESSON 10: SELF-ASSESSMENT #5

CAPTURING AND RECORDING YOUR INITIAL NUMBERS: THE SUPER 6 & SEATED WHOLE BODY MENU

Reflection:

- How did that menu make you feel - were you short of breath? If you were short of breath, were you doing Flow-Controlled Breathing© or possibly going through the exercises too fast?
- What muscles did you feel working?
- Was it challenging?
- Were some exercises harder than others and if so, which ones?
- How did your oxygen saturation and heart rate compare before, during, and after exercise?
- What has improved? Can you feel these improvements?
- When you go to do this menu again in the future, what are some of your goals?

Please record your responses to the above questions in the space below.

LESSON 10: SELF-ASSESSMENT #5

CAPTURING AND RECORDING YOUR INITIAL NUMBERS: THE SUPER 6 & SEATED WHOLE BODY MENU

After completing the **Super 6**, use the **Shortness of Breath Scale** below to quantify your shortness of breath by circling the column containing the shortness of breath number that best describes how you feel.

***If you need a refresher on what this scale is and how to use it, please reference the video in Section 2 Lesson 4 entitled "Introduction to the Shortness of Breath Scale".*

Shortness of Breath Scale

SOB #	0	½	1	2	3	4	5	6	7	8
SEVERITY	NONE	JUST NOTICEABLE	VERY SLIGHT	SLIGHT	MODERATE	MORE MODERATE	SEVERE	MORE SEVERE	VERY SEVERE	MAXIMUM
	Normal Speech				Choppy Speech		Can't Speak		Call 911!	

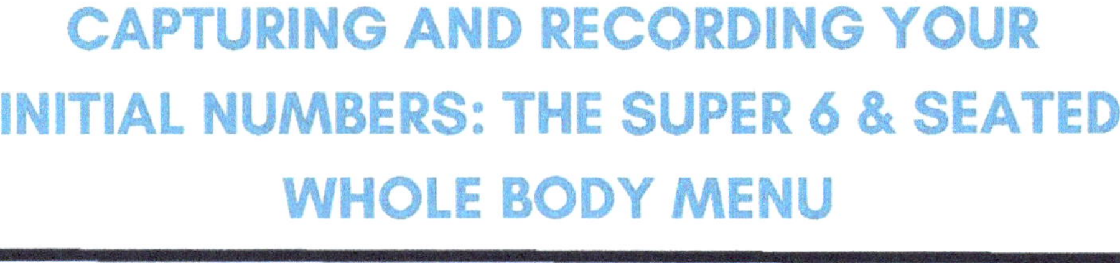
CAPTURING AND RECORDING YOUR INITIAL NUMBERS: THE SUPER 6 & SEATED WHOLE BODY MENU

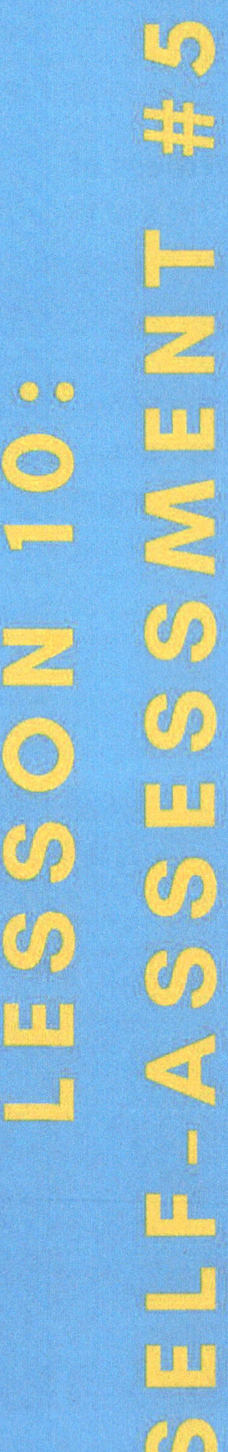
LESSON 10:
SELF-ASSESSMENT #5

After completing the **Super 6**, use the **Work Scale** below to quantify the amount of work you performed completing these exercises by circling the column containing the work number that best describes how you feel. You may designate a number for each exercise or choose a number that best represents the amount of work performed throughout the entire menu.

***If you need a refresher on what this scale is and how to use it, please reference the video in Section 3 Lesson 4 entitled "Introduction to the Work Scale".*

How difficult is the exercise that you are doing right now?

This is no work at all	Not bad at all, but too easy	A little harder, but still good	This is good, I'm challenged	Getting too difficult	Nope, can't do it
0	1	2	3	4	5

Let's try and stay between 2 and 3.5

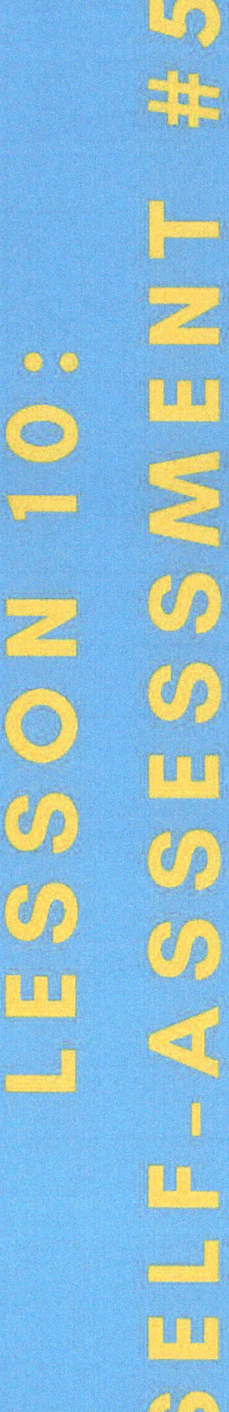

CAPTURING AND RECORDING YOUR INITIAL NUMBERS: THE SUPER 6 & SEATED WHOLE BODY MENU

To-Do:

After watching the explanation of the **Seated Whole Body Menu** and familiarizing yourself with the exercises by looking at the chart as well as watching the step-by-step exercise guide for this menu, begin doing the exercises in the order they appear both in the aforementioned chart and video.

Be sure to take rests when you are feeling short of breath as well as between each exercise as needed. Check and record your oxygen saturation and heart rate using your pulse oximeter both before, during, and after exercising. Please record these numbers in the tables on the next page.

As a reminder, put the pulse oximeter on your finger and wait about 20 seconds to allow the device to capture the most accurate readings. If you find that your oxygen saturation and heart rate readings are much different than your normal readings, please put the device on your other hand, trying multiple fingers until you get the best signal strength and reading.

Try your best to capture 2-3 oxygen saturation and heart rate readings from your pulse oximeter ***DURING*** the time you are walking and separate each below in the appropriate box with commas. Lastly but certainly not least, **remember to do your Flow-Controlled Breathing©!**

As a reminder, please check your oxygen saturation and heart rate readings frequently during this exercise. If you find that your oxygen saturation drops below or your heart rate goes above the accepted values your healthcare providers gave to you, immediately stop.

Reminder: I usually recommend maintaining an oxygen saturation of 92% or higher.

LESSON 10:
SELF-ASSESSMENT #5

CAPTURING AND RECORDING YOUR INITIAL NUMBERS: THE SUPER 6 & SEATED WHOLE BODY MENU

Pulse Oximeter Reading (Before exercise)

Oxygen Saturation (%)	
Heart Rate (bpm)	
Supplemental Oxygen (L) (if you don't wear oxygen, write "room air")	

Pulse Oximeter Reading (During exercise; multiple readings separated by commas)

Oxygen Saturation (%)	
Heart Rate (bpm)	
Supplemental Oxygen (L) (if you don't wear oxygen, write "room air")	
Number of rests	

Pulse Oximeter Reading (After exercise)

Oxygen Saturation (%)	
Heart Rate (bpm)	
Supplemental Oxygen (L) (if you don't wear oxygen, write "room air")	

LESSON 10: SELF-ASSESSMENT #5

CAPTURING AND RECORDING YOUR INITIAL NUMBERS: THE SUPER 6 & SEATED WHOLE BODY MENU

Reflection:

- How did that menu make you feel - were you short of breath? If you were short of breath, were you doing Flow-Controlled Breathing© or possibly going through the exercises too fast?
- What muscles did you feel working?
- Was it challenging?
- Were some exercises harder than others and if so, which ones?
- How did your oxygen saturation and heart rate compare before, during, and after exercise?
- What has improved? Can you feel these improvements?
- When you go to do this menu again in the future, what are some of your goals?

Please record your responses to the above questions in the space below.

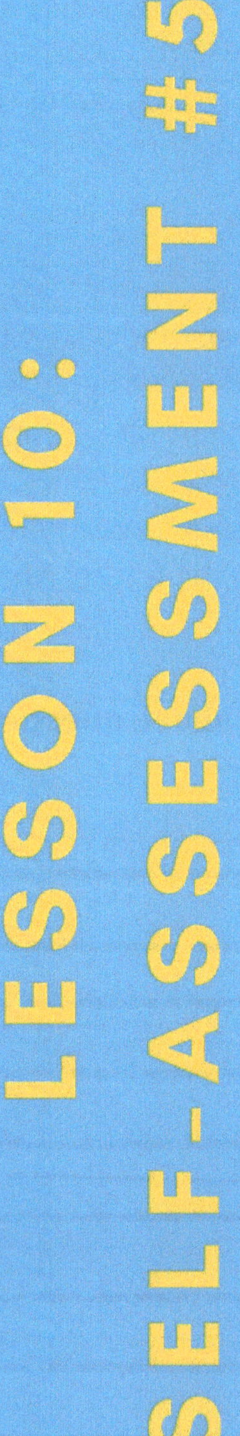

CAPTURING AND RECORDING YOUR INITIAL NUMBERS: THE SUPER 6 & SEATED WHOLE BODY MENU

After completing the **Seated Whole Body Menu**, use the **Shortness of Breath Scale** below to quantify your shortness of breath by circling the column containing the shortness of breath number that best describes how you feel.

***If you need a refresher on what this scale is and how to use it, please reference the video in Section 2 Lesson 4 entitled "Introduction to the Shortness of Breath Scale".*

Shortness of Breath Scale

SOB #	0	½	1	2	3	4	5	6	7	8
SEVERITY	NONE	JUST NOTICEABLE	VERY SLIGHT	SLIGHT	MODERATE	MORE MODERATE	SEVERE	MORE SEVERE	VERY SEVERE	MAXIMUM
	Normal Speech				Choppy Speech		Can't Speak		Call 911!	

LESSON 10:
SELF-ASSESSMENT #5

CAPTURING AND RECORDING YOUR INITIAL NUMBERS: THE SUPER 6 & SEATED WHOLE BODY MENU

Reflection:

Take a few minutes and compare the shortness of breath number you chose after **Super 6 (Self-Assessment #5 page 101)** versus the one you chose after the **Seated Whole Body Menu** above. Which number is higher? Does the higher number reflect the menu that you felt was more difficult?

We ideally want you to be breathing at a **2-3** on this **Shortness of Breath Scale**, did you remain within this range during both exercises menus? If not, reflect on why your shortness of breath selection may have been above or below this range (i.e. consider your pace and your proper use of the Flow-Controlled Breathing© technique).

Also, please keep in mind that your shortness of breath selection for these menus may differ as one menu is done sitting while the other is done standing. As you continue to progress through this course you will get stronger and have decreased shortness of breath, allowing you to successfully complete exercises that you were not able to do before. Keep up the good work!

Please record your responses to the above questions in the space below.

LESSON 10: SELF-ASSESSMENT #5

CAPTURING AND RECORDING YOUR INITIAL NUMBERS: THE SUPER 6 & SEATED WHOLE BODY MENU

After completing the **Seated Whole Body Menu**, use the **Work Scale** below to quantify the amount of work you performed completing these exercises by circling the column containing the work number that best describes how you feel. You may designate a number for each exercise or choose a number that best represents the amount of work performed throughout the entire menu.

***If you need a refresher on what this scale is and how to use it, please reference the video in Section 3 Lesson 4 entitled "Introduction to the Work Scale".*

How difficult is the exercise that you are doing right now?

This is no work at all	Not bad at all, but too easy	A little harder, but still good	This is good, I'm challenged	Getting too difficult	Nope, can't do it
0	1	2	3	4	5

<u>Let's try and stay between 2 and 3.5</u>

LESSON 10: SELF-ASSESSMENT #5

CAPTURING AND RECORDING YOUR INITIAL NUMBERS: THE SUPER 6 & SEATED WHOLE BODY MENU

Reflection:

Take a few minutes and compare the work number you chose after the **Super 6 (page 102)** versus the one you chose after the the **Seated Whole Body Menu** above. Which number is higher? Does the higher number reflect the menu that you felt was more difficult?

We ideally want you to be breathing at a **2-3.5** on this **Work Scale**, did you remain within this range during both exercises menus? If not, reflect on why your work selection may have been above or below this range (i.e. going too slow and/or fast, not using the Flow-Controlled Breathing© technique, using too heavy of a weight, doing too many repetitions, etc.).

Also, please keep in mind that your work scale selections for these menus may differ as one menu is done sitting while the other is done standing. As you continue to progress through this course you will get stronger and your work scale number will decrease, allowing you to successfully complete exercises that you were not able to do before. Keep up the good work!

Please record your responses to the above questions in the space below.

LESSON 10: SELF-ASSESMENT #5

CAPTURING AND RECORDING YOUR INITIAL NUMBERS: THE SUPER 6 & SEATED WHOLE BODY MENU

Reflection:

Take a few minutes to reflect on your experience doing the **Super 6** and the **Seated Whole Body Menu**.

- Was one menu more difficult than the other?
- How was your balance?
- How did these menus compare to your experience doing **Suki's Seated Power Menu** and the **Core 4**?
- Compare your oxygen saturation and heart rate before, during, and after for the **Super 6** and the **Seated Whole Body Menu.**
- What has improved? Can you feel these improvements?
- Write down any goals you have for yourself after completing these menus.

If you did have trouble with either of these menus, it is ok--as you progress through this program, you will get stronger, your balance will improve, and overall these exercises will become easier!

Please record your responses to the above questions in the space below.

Great job, you've completed your fifth assessment! Make sure that all the above information is filled out and keep this assessment in a safe place.

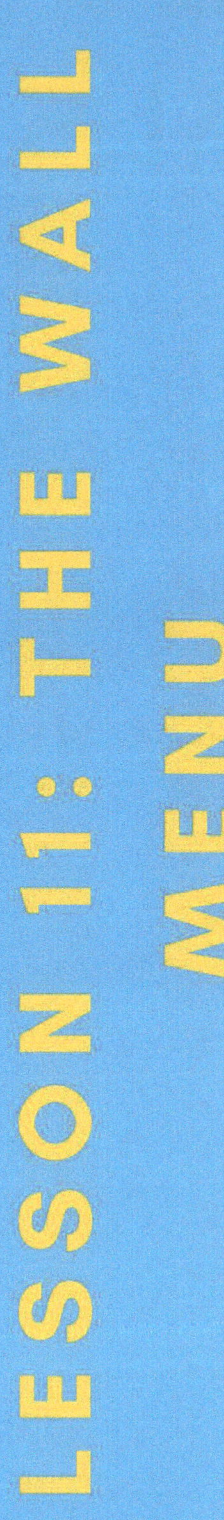

Objectives:

I. To use the wall as a flat reference point to restack your load bearing joints.

II. To open your chest cavity to allow for easier breathing and chest expansion.

III. Rotate the heads of the humerus to reeducate proper shoulder movement.

IV. Isolate upper and lower body muscles that normally don't engage due to compensation.

V. Use the **Shortness of Breath Scale** to quantify your shortness of breath after completing the **Wall Menu.**

VI. Use the **Work Scale** to quantify the amount of work being done during the **Wall Menu.**

To-Do:

Watch the "What is the Wall Menu" video, take notes below as needed. ☐

LESSON 11: WALL MENU

REQUIRED MATERIALS

- ☑ PULSE OXIMETER
- ☑ SUPPLEMENTAL OXYGEN, IF PRESCRIBED
- ☑ TIMER
- ☑ STRAIGHT WALL
- ☑ TOWEL ROLL
- ☑ ITEM FOR SUPPORT (I.E. CHAIR, LOCKED ROLLING WALKER)
- ☑ WATER (GLASS OR BOTTLE)

LESSON 11: WALL MENU

To-Do:

- [ ] Look at chart of exercises, including sets and set/time. Familiarize yourself with exercise names.
- [ ] Watch the "Menu #5: The Wall Menu" video, take notes below as needed.

Important Reminders:

1) Proper posture [squared feet, pinched shoulders, level chin, no leaning]

2) Blow & Lift while doing Flow-Controlled Breathing©

3) Go slowly

4) Stop when winded

5) Have fun! You're **not** just exercising, *you're working towards your goal!*

Assignment:

Now it is time to begin practicing this menu. Feel free to have the exercise video playing to help guide you. Use **Self-Assessment #6** beginning on **page 119** to record your numbers and answer the corresponding questions.

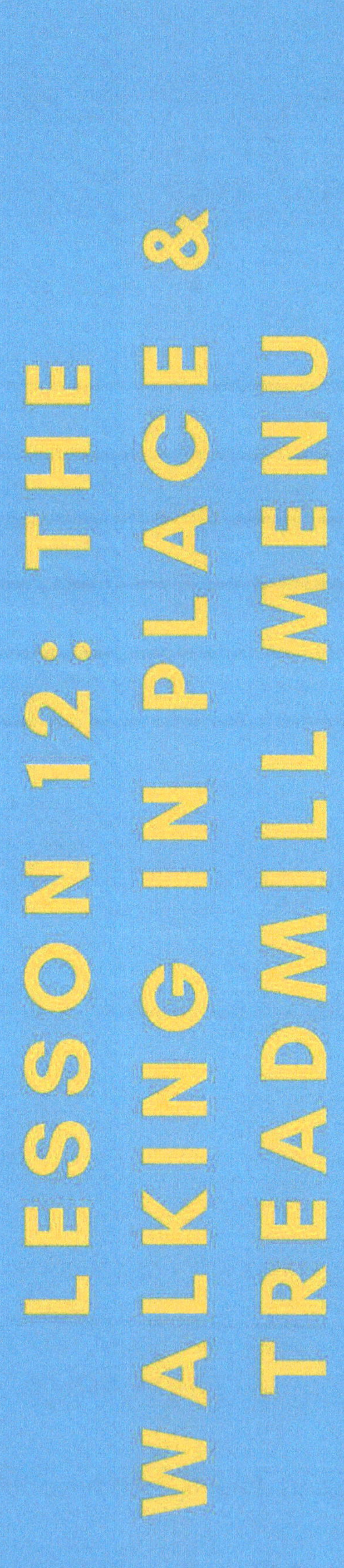

Objectives:

I. Build stamina, endurance, and strength while also improving your breathing doing our main mode of transportation... walking.

II. Use the **Shortness of Breath Scale** to quantify your shortness of breath after completing the **Walking in Place & Treadmill Menu.**

III. Use the **Work Scale** to quantify the amount of work being done during the **Walking in Place & Treadmill Menu.**

To-Do:

Watch the "What is the Walking in Place & Treadmill Menu" video, take notes below as needed. ☐

LESSON 12: THE WALKING IN PLACE MENU

REQUIRED MATERIALS

- ☑ PULSE OXIMETER
- ☑ SUPPLEMENTAL OXYGEN, IF PRESCRIBED
- ☑ WATER (GLASS OR BOTTLE)

LESSON 12: THE TREADMILL MENU

REQUIRED MATERIALS

- ☑ PULSE OXIMETER
- ☑ SUPPLEMENTAL OXYGEN, IF PRESCRIBED
- ☑ TIMER
- ☑ TREADMILL
- ☑ WATER (GLASS OR BOTTLE)

LESSON 12: THE WALKING IN PLACE & TREADMILL MENU

To-Do:

- [ ] *Regardless of if you have access to a treadmill or not,* watch the "Menu #6: Walking in Place" video, take notes below as needed.

- [ ] *If you have access to a treadmill*, watch the "Menu #6: Treadmill" video, take notes below as needed.

Important Reminders:

1) Proper posture [squared feet, pinched shoulders, level chin, no leaning]

2) Blow & Lift while doing Flow-Controlled Breathing©

3) Go slowly

4) Stop when winded

5) Have fun! You're **not** just exercising, *you're working towards your goal!*

Assignment:

Now it is time to begin practicing this menu. Feel free to have the exercise video playing to help guide you. Use **Self-Assessment #6** beginning on **page 125** to record your numbers and answer the corresponding questions.

LESSON 13: INTRODUCTION TO SELF-ASSESSMENT #6

Objectives:

I. Understand the purpose and contents of **Self-Assessment #6**

II. Understand how to use **Self-Assessment #6.**

To-Do:

Watch the "Introduction to Self-Assessment #6" video, take notes below as needed. ☐

Assignment:

Before continuing on to complete **Self-Assessment #6**, please take some time to continue to familiarize yourself with **Self-Assessment #6** by flipping through the next 15 pages in this workbook. Take notes below as needed.

LESSON 13: SELF-ASSESSMENT #6

CAPTURING AND RECORDING YOUR INITIAL NUMBERS: WALL MENU & WALKING IN PLACE & TREADMILL MENU

Objectives:

I. Provides an opportunity to reflect on the **Wall Menu** and the **Walking in Place & Treadmill Menu** and to quantitatively compare your oxygen saturation and heart rate during various exercises in these menus.

II. Provides a reference point when comparing oxygen saturation and heart rate at this point in the program in comparison to other checkpoints in the program to quantify your progress.

III. Provides **quantification** of shortness of breath after the **Wall Menu** and the **Walking in Place & Treadmill Menu** using the **Shortness of Breath Scale**.

IV. Provides a **quantitative comparison** of shortness of breath after the **Wall Menu** and the **Walking in Place & Treadmill Menu** using the **Shortness of Breath Scale**.

V. Provides **quantification** of the amount of work being performed after the **Wall Menu** and the **Walking in Place & Treadmill Menu** using the **Work Scale**.

VI. Provides a **quantitative comparison** of the amount of work being performed after the **Wall Menu** and the **Walking in Place & Treadmill Menu** using the **Work Scale**.

LESSON 13:
SELF-ASSESSMENT #6

CAPTURING AND RECORDING YOUR INITIAL NUMBERS: WALL MENU & WALKING IN PLACE & TREADMILL MENU

To-Do:

After watching the explanation of the **Wall Menu** and familiarizing yourself with the exercises by looking at the chart as well as watching the step-by-step exercise guide for this menu, begin doing the exercises in the order they appear both in the aforementioned chart and video.

Be sure to take rests when you are feeling short of breath as well as between each exercise as needed. Check and record your oxygen saturation and heart rate using your pulse oximeter both before, during, and after exercising. Please record these numbers in the tables on the next page.

As a reminder, put the pulse oximeter on your finger and wait about 20 seconds to allow the device to capture the most accurate readings. If you find that your oxygen saturation and heart rate readings are much different than your normal readings, please put the device on your other hand, trying multiple fingers until you get the best signal strength and reading.
Try your best to capture 2-3 oxygen saturation and heart rate readings from your pulse oximeter ***DURING*** the time you are walking and separate each below in the appropriate box with commas. Lastly but certainly not least, **remember to do your Flow-Controlled Breathing©**!

As a reminder, please check your oxygen saturation and heart rate readings frequently during this exercise. If you find that your oxygen saturation drops below or your heart rate goes above the accepted values your healthcare providers gave to you, immediately stop.

Reminder: I usually recommend maintaining an oxygen saturation of 92% or higher.

LESSON 13:
SELF-ASSESSMENT #6

CAPTURING AND RECORDING YOUR INITIAL NUMBERS: WALL MENU & WALKING IN PLACE & TREADMILL MENU

Pulse Oximeter Reading (Before exercise)

Oxygen Saturation (%)	
Heart Rate (bpm)	
Supplemental Oxygen (L) *(if you don't wear oxygen, write "room air")*	

Pulse Oximeter Reading
(During exercise; multiple readings separated by commas)

Oxygen Saturation (%)	
Heart Rate (bpm)	
Supplemental Oxygen (L) *(if you don't wear oxygen, write "room air")*	
Number of rests	

Pulse Oximeter Reading (After exercise)

Oxygen Saturation (%)	
Heart Rate (bpm)	
Supplemental Oxygen (L) *(if you don't wear oxygen, write "room air")*	

CAPTURING AND RECORDING YOUR INITIAL NUMBERS: WALL MENU & WALKING IN PLACE & TREADMILL MENU

Reflection:

- How did that menu make you feel - were you short of breath? If you were short of breath, were you doing Flow-Controlled Breathing© or possibly going through the exercises too fast?
- What muscles did you feel working?
- Was it challenging?
- Were some exercises harder than others and if so, which ones?
- How did your oxygen saturation and heart rate compare before, during, and after exercise?
- What has improved? Can you feel these improvements?
- When you go to do this menu again in the future, what are some of your goals?

Please record your responses to the above questions in the space below.

LESSON 13: SELF-ASSESSMENT #6

CAPTURING AND RECORDING YOUR INITIAL NUMBERS: WALL MENU & WALKING IN PLACE & TREADMILL MENU

After completing the **Wall Menu**, use the **Shortness of Breath Scale** below to quantify your shortness of breath by circling the column containing the shortness of breath number that best describes how you feel.

***If you need a refresher on what this scale is and how to use it, please reference the video in Section 2 Lesson 4 entitled "Introduction to the Shortness of Breath Scale".*

Shortness of Breath Scale

SOB #	0	½	1	2	3	4	5	6	7	8
SEVERITY	NONE	JUST NOTICEABLE	VERY SLIGHT	SLIGHT	MODERATE	MORE MODERATE	SEVERE	MORE SEVERE	VERY SEVERE	MAXIMUM
	Normal Speech				Choppy Speech		Can't Speak		Call 911!	

LESSON 13:
SELF-ASSESSMENT #6

CAPTURING AND RECORDING YOUR INITIAL NUMBERS: WALL MENU & WALKING IN PLACE & TREADMILL MENU

After completing the **Wall Menu**, use the **Work Scale** below to quantify the amount of work you performed completing these exercises by circling the column containing the work number that best describes how you feel. You may designate a number for each exercise or choose a number that best represents the amount of work performed throughout the entire menu.

***If you need a refresher on what this scale is and how to use it, please reference the video in Section 3 Lesson 4 entitled "Introduction to the Work Scale".*

How difficult is the exercise that you are doing right now?

This is no work at all	Not bad at all, but too easy	A little harder, but still good	This is good, I'm challenged	Getting too difficult	Nope, can't do it
0	1	2	3	4	5

Let's try and stay between 2 and 3.5

LESSON 13: SELF-ASSESSMENT #6

CAPTURING AND RECORDING YOUR INITIAL NUMBERS: WALL MENU & WALKING IN PLACE & TREADMILL MENU

To-Do:

After watching the explanation of the **Walking in Place & Treadmill Menu** and watching the instructional video for the **Walking in Place** portion of this menu, begin practicing this exercise.

Be sure to take rests when you are feeling short of breath. Check and record your oxygen saturation and heart rate using your pulse oximeter both before, during, and after exercising. Please record these numbers in the tables on the next page.

As a reminder, put the pulse oximeter on your finger and wait about 20 seconds to allow the device to capture the most accurate readings. If you find that your oxygen saturation and heart rate readings are much different than your normal readings, please put the device on your other hand, trying multiple fingers until you get the best signal strength and reading.

Try your best to capture 2-3 oxygen saturation and heart rate readings from your pulse oximeter ***DURING*** the time you are walking in place and separate each below in the appropriate box with commas. Lastly but certainly not least, **remember to do your Flow-Controlled Breathing©!**

As a reminder, please check your oxygen saturation and heart rate readings frequently during this exercise. If you find that your oxygen saturation drops below or your heart rate goes above the accepted values your healthcare providers gave to you, immediately stop.

Reminder: I usually recommend maintaining an oxygen saturation 92% or higher.

LESSON 13: SELF-ASSESSMENT #6

CAPTURING AND RECORDING YOUR INITIAL NUMBERS: WALL MENU & WALKING IN PLACE & TREADMILL MENU

Pulse Oximeter Reading (Before exercise)

Oxygen Saturation (%)	
Heart Rate (bpm)	
Supplemental Oxygen (L) (if you don't wear oxygen, write "room air")	

Pulse Oximeter Reading
(During exercise; multiple readings separated by commas)

Oxygen Saturation (%)	
Heart Rate (bpm)	
Supplemental Oxygen (L) (if you don't wear oxygen, write "room air")	
Number of rests	

Pulse Oximeter Reading (After exercise)

Oxygen Saturation (%)	
Heart Rate (bpm)	
Supplemental Oxygen (L) (if you don't wear oxygen, write "room air")	

LESSON 13: SELF-ASSESSMENT #6

CAPTURING AND RECORDING YOUR INITIAL NUMBERS: WALL MENU & WALKING IN PLACE & TREADMILL MENU

Reflection:

- How did that menu make you feel - were you short of breath? If you were short of breath, were you doing Flow-Controlled Breathing© or possibly going through the exercises too fast?
- What muscles did you feel working?
- Was it challenging?
- Were some exercises harder than others and if so, which ones?
- How did your oxygen saturation and heart rate compare before, during, and after exercise?
- What has improved? Can you feel these improvements?
- When you go to do this menu again in the future, what are some of your goals?

Please record your responses to the above questions in the space below.

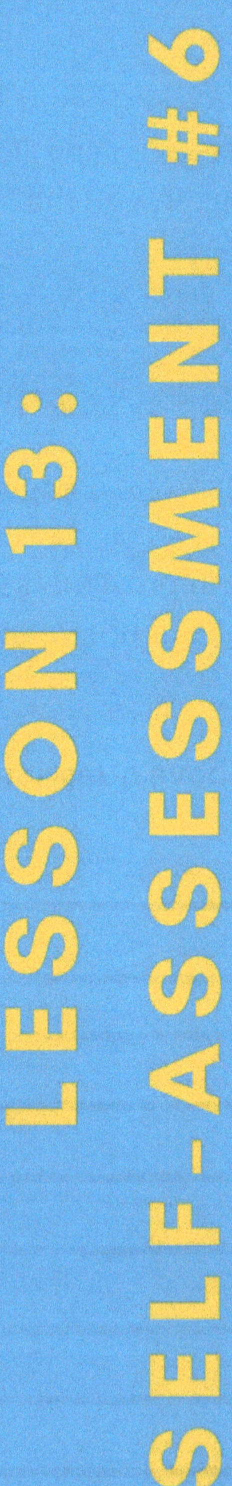

CAPTURING AND RECORDING YOUR INITIAL NUMBERS: WALL MENU & WALKING IN PLACE & TREADMILL MENU

After completing the **Walking in Place** portion of the **Walking in Place & Treadmill Menu**, use the **Shortness of Breath Scale** below to quantify your shortness of breath by circling the column containing the shortness of breath number that best describes how you feel.

***If you need a refresher on what this scale is and how to use it, please reference the video in Section 2 Lesson 4 entitled "Introduction to the Shortness of Breath Scale".*

Shortness of Breath Scale

SOB #	0	½	1	2	3	4	5	6	7	8
SEVERITY	NONE	JUST NOTICEABLE	VERY SLIGHT	SLIGHT	MODERATE	MORE MODERATE	SEVERE	MORE SEVERE	VERY SEVERE	MAXIMUM
	Normal Speech				Choppy Speech		Can't Speak		Call 911!	

CAPTURING AND RECORDING YOUR INITIAL NUMBERS: WALL MENU & WALKING IN PLACE & TREADMILL MENU

Reflection:

Take a few minutes and compare the shortness of breath number you chose after **Wall Menu (Self-Assessment #6 page 123)** versus the one you chose after the **Walking in Place** portion of the **Walking in Place & Treadmill Menu** above. Which number is higher? Does the higher number reflect the menu that you felt was more difficult?

We ideally want you to be breathing at a **2-3** on this **Shortness of Breath Scale**, did you remain within this range during both exercises menus? If not, reflect on why your shortness of breath selection may have been above or below this range (i.e. consider your pace and your proper use of the Flow-Controlled Breathing© technique).

Also, please keep in mind that your shortness of breath selection for these menus may differ as one menu is done sitting while the other is done standing. As you continue to progress through this course you will get stronger and have decreased shortness of breath, allowing you to successfully complete exercises that you were not able to do before. Keep up the good work!

Please record your responses to the above questions in the space below.

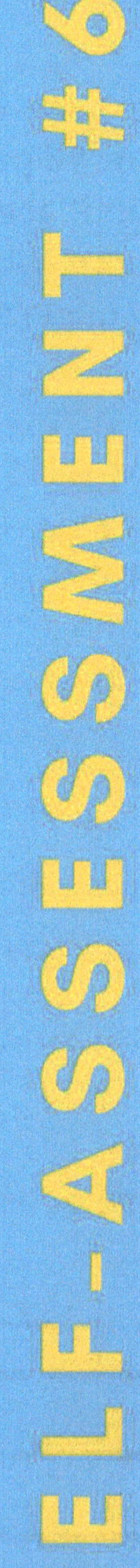

CAPTURING AND RECORDING YOUR INITIAL NUMBERS: WALL MENU & WALKING IN PLACE & TREADMILL MENU

After completing the **Walking in Place** portion of the **Walking in Place & Treadmill Menu**, use the **Work Scale** below to quantify the amount of work you performed completing these exercises by circling the column containing the work number that best describes how you feel. You may designate a number for each exercise or choose a number that best represents the amount of work performed throughout the entire menu.

***If you need a refresher on what this scale is and how to use it, please reference the video in Section 3 Lesson 4 entitled "Introduction to the Work Scale".*

How difficult is the exercise that you are doing right now?

This is no work at all	Not bad at all, but too easy	A little harder, but still good	This is good, I'm challenged	Getting too difficult	Nope, can't do it
0	1	2	3	4	5

Let's try and stay between 2 and 3.5

LESSON 13: SELF-ASSESSMENT #6

CAPTURING AND RECORDING YOUR INITIAL NUMBERS: WALL MENU & WALKING IN PLACE & TREADMILL MENU

Reflection:

Take a few minutes and compare the work number you chose after the **Wall Menu (page 124)** versus the one you chose after the **Walking in Place** portion of the **Walking in Place & Treadmill Menu** above. Which number is higher? Does the higher number reflect the menu that you felt was more difficult?

We ideally want you to be breathing at a **2-3.5** on this **Work Scale**, did you remain within this range during both exercises menus? If not, reflect on why your work selection may have been above or below this range (i.e. going too slow and/or fast, not using the Flow-Controlled Breathing© technique, using too heavy of a weight, doing too many repetitions, etc.).

Also, please keep in mind that your work scale selections for these menus may differ as one menu is done sitting while the other is done standing. As you continue to progress through this course you will get stronger and your work scale number will decrease, allowing you to successfully complete exercises that you were not able to do before. Keep up the good work!

Please record your responses to the above questions in the space below.

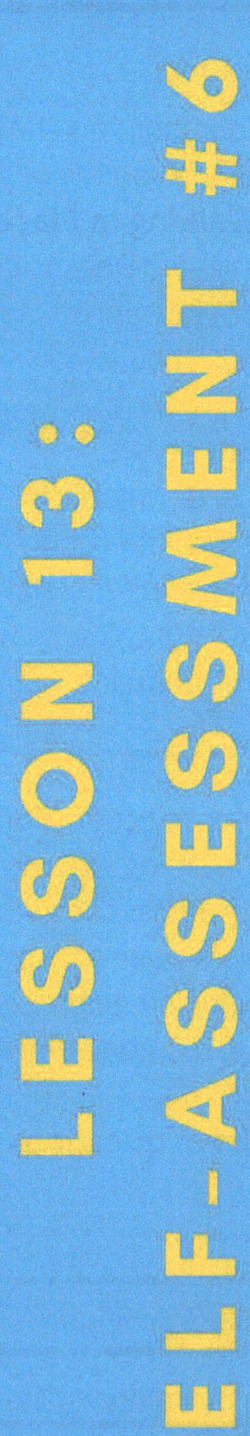

CAPTURING AND RECORDING YOUR INITIAL NUMBERS: WALL MENU & WALKING IN PLACE & TREADMILL MENU

To-Do:

If you have access to a treadmill, please continue on with this portion of the self-assessment.

If you do not have access to a treadmill, please skip to page 143 of this self-assessment.

After watching the explanation of the **Walking in Place & Treadmill Menu** and watching the instructional video for the **Treadmill** portion of this menu, begin practicing this exercise.

Be sure to take rests when you are feeling short of breath. Check and record your oxygen saturation and heart rate using your pulse oximeter both before, during, and after exercising. Please record these numbers in the tables on the next page.

As a reminder, put the pulse oximeter on your finger and wait about 20 seconds to allow the device to capture the most accurate readings. If you find that your oxygen saturation and heart rate readings are much different than your normal readings, please put the device on your other hand, trying multiple fingers until you get the best signal strength and reading.

Try your best to capture 2-3 oxygen saturation and heart rate readings from your pulse oximeter ***DURING*** the time you are walking in place and separate each below in the appropriate box with commas. Lastly but certainly not least, **remember to do your Flow-Controlled Breathing©!**

LESSON 13: SELF-ASSESSMENT #6

CAPTURING AND RECORDING YOUR INITIAL NUMBERS: WALL MENU & WALKING IN PLACE & TREADMILL MENU

As a reminder, please check your oxygen saturation and heart rate readings frequently during this exercise. If you find that your oxygen saturation drops below or your heart rate goes above the accepted values your healthcare providers gave to you, immediately stop.

Reminder: I usually recommend maintaining an oxygen saturation of 92% or higher.

Pulse Oximeter Reading (Before exercise)

Oxygen Saturation (%)	
Heart Rate (bpm)	
Supplemental Oxygen (L) *(if you don't wear oxygen, write "room air")*	

Pulse Oximeter Reading
(During exercise; multiple readings separated by commas)

Oxygen Saturation (%)	
Heart Rate (bpm)	
Supplemental Oxygen (L) *(if you don't wear oxygen, write "room air")*	
Number of rests	

Pulse Oximeter Reading (After exercise)

Oxygen Saturation (%)	
Heart Rate (bpm)	
Supplemental Oxygen (L) *(if you don't wear oxygen, write "room air")*	

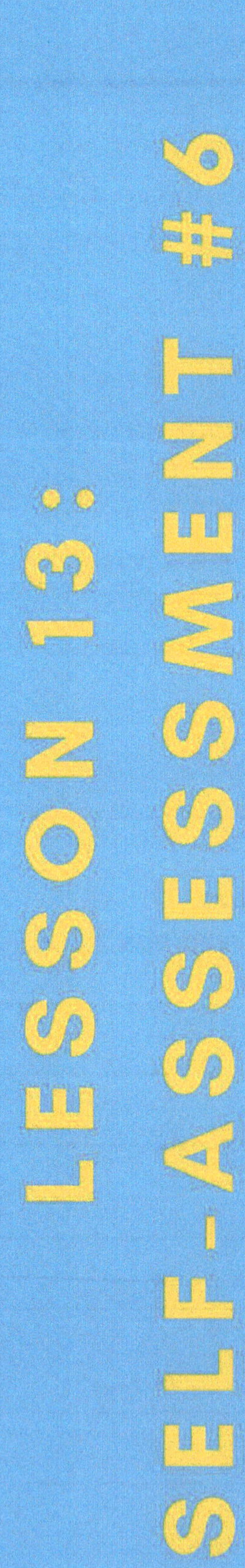

CAPTURING AND RECORDING YOUR INITIAL NUMBERS: WALL MENU & WALKING IN PLACE & TREADMILL MENU

Reflection:

- How did that menu make you feel - were you short of breath? If you were short of breath, were you doing Flow-Controlled Breathing© or possibly going through the exercises too fast?
- What muscles did you feel working?
- Was it challenging?
- Were some exercises harder than others and if so, which ones?
- How did your oxygen saturation and heart rate compare before, during, and after exercise?
- What has improved? Can you feel these improvements?
- When you go to do this menu again in the future, what are some of your goals?

Please record your responses to the above questions in the space below.

LESSON 13:
SELF-ASSESSMENT #6

CAPTURING AND RECORDING YOUR INITIAL NUMBERS: WALL MENU & WALKING IN PLACE & TREADMILL MENU

After completing the **Treadmill** portion of the **Walking in Place & Treadmill Menu**, use the **Shortness of Breath Scale** below to quantify your shortness of breath by circling the column containing the shortness of breath number that best describes how you feel.

***If you need a refresher on what this scale is and how to use it, please reference the video in Section 2 Lesson 4 entitled "Introduction to the Shortness of Breath Scale".*

Shortness of Breath Scale

SOB #	0	½	1	2	3	4	5	6	7	8
SEVERITY	NONE	JUST NOTICEABLE	VERY SLIGHT	SLIGHT	MODERATE	MORE MODERATE	SEVERE	MORE SEVERE	VERY SEVERE	MAXIMUM
	Normal Speech				Choppy Speech		Can't Speak		Call 911!	

LESSON 13: SELF-ASSESSMENT #6

CAPTURING AND RECORDING YOUR INITIAL NUMBERS: WALL MENU & WALKING IN PLACE & TREADMILL MENU

Reflection:

Take a few minutes and compare the shortness of breath number you chose after **Wall Menu (page 123)** versus the one you chose after the **Treadmill** portion of the **Walking in Place & Treadmill Menu** above. Which number is higher? Does the higher number reflect the menu that you felt was more difficult?

We ideally want you to be breathing at a **2-3** on this **Shortness of Breath Scale**, did you remain within this range during both exercises menus? If not, reflect on why your shortness of breath selection may have been above or below this range (i.e. consider your pace and your proper use of the Flow-Controlled Breathing© technique).

Also, please keep in mind that your shortness of breath selection for these menus may differ as one menu is done sitting while the other is done standing. As you continue to progress through this course you will get stronger and have decreased shortness of breath, allowing you to successfully complete exercises that you were not able to do before. Keep up the good work!

Please record your responses to the above questions in the space below.

LESSON 13:
SELF-ASSESSMENT #6

CAPTURING AND RECORDING YOUR INITIAL NUMBERS: WALL MENU & WALKING IN PLACE & TREADMILL MENU

After completing the **Treadmill** portion of the **Walking in Place & Treadmill Menu**, use the **Work Scale** below to quantify the amount of work you performed completing these exercises by circling the column containing the work number that best describes how you feel. You may designate a number for each exercise or choose a number that best represents the amount of work performed throughout the entire menu.

***If you need a refresher on what this scale is and how to use it, please reference the video in Section 3 Lesson 4 entitled "Introduction to the Work Scale".*

How difficult is the exercise that you are doing right now?

This is no work at all	Not bad at all, but too easy	A little harder, but still good	This is good, I'm challenged	Getting too difficult	Nope, can't do it
0	1	2	3	4	5

<u>Let's try and stay between 2 and 3.5</u>

LESSON 13: SELF-ASSESSMENT #6

CAPTURING AND RECORDING YOUR INITIAL NUMBERS: WALL MENU & WALKING IN PLACE & TREADMILL MENU

Reflection:

Take a few minutes and compare the work number you chose after the **Wall Menu (page 124)** versus the one you chose after the **Treadmill** portion of the **Walking in Place & Treadmill Menu** above. Which number is higher? Does the higher number reflect the menu that you felt was more difficult?

We ideally want you to be breathing at a **2-3.5** on this **Work Scale**, did you remain within this range during both exercises menus? If not, reflect on why your work selection may have been above or below this range (i.e. going too slow and/or fast, not using the Flow-Controlled Breathing© technique, using too heavy of a weight, doing too many repetitions, etc.).

Also, please keep in mind that your work scale selections for these menus may differ as one menu is done sitting while the other is done standing. As you continue to progress through this course you will get stronger and your work scale number will decrease, allowing you to successfully complete exercises that you were not able to do before. Keep up the good work!

Please record your responses to the above questions in the space below.

LESSON 13: SELF-ASSESSMENT #6

CAPTURING AND RECORDING YOUR INITIAL NUMBERS: WALL MENU & WALKING IN PLACE & TREADMILL MENU

Reflection:

Take a few minutes to reflect on your experience doing the **Wall Menu** and the **Walking in Place & Treadmill Menu.**

- Was one menu more difficult than the other?
- How was your balance?
- How did these menus compare to your experience doing **Suki's Seated Power Menu,** the **Core 4,** the **Super 6,** and the **Seated Whole Body Menu**?
- Compare your oxygen saturation and heart rate before, during, and after for the **Wall Menu** and the **Walking in Place & Treadmill Menu**.
- What has improved? Can you feel these improvements?
- Write down any goals you have for yourself after completing these menus.

If you did have trouble with either of these menus, it is okay - as you progress through this program, you will get stronger, your balance will improve, and overall these exercises will become easier!

Please record your responses to the above questions in the space below.

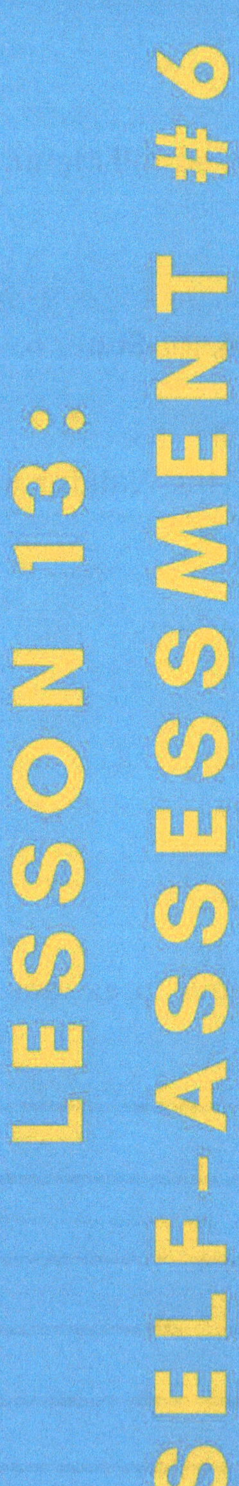

CAPTURING AND RECORDING YOUR INITIAL NUMBERS: WALL MENU & WALKING IN PLACE & TREADMILL MENU

Reflection:

Take a few minutes to look at your oxygen saturation and heart rate from the previous Self-Assessments #1-5. Please also reflect on physical, emotional, and psychological improvements that you feel as well.

- What changes and improvements do you notice (ex. increase in strength, decrease in anxiety, elevated mood, better balance)? How does it make you feel to see these improvements?
- What are some goals you have for yourself moving forward with these exercises and the program?
- Now that you see these improvements, how will this change your daily life and the lives of your loved ones?
- What activities will you now try that you couldn't do before you started this program?

Please record your responses to the above questions in the space below.

Great job, you've completed your sixth and final assessment! Make sure that all the above information is filled out and please keep this assessment in a safe place.

Section 5

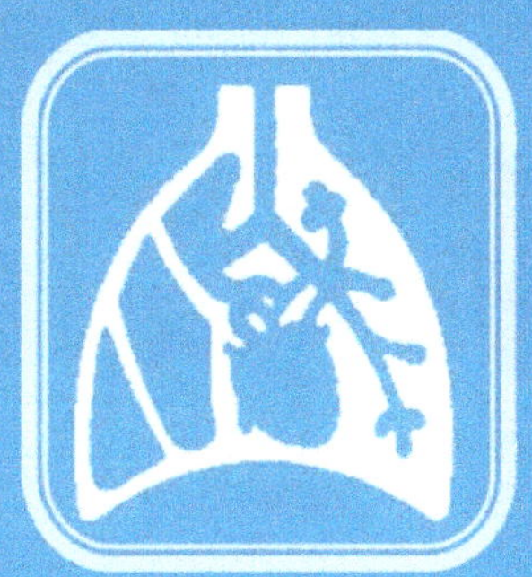

THOUGHT OF THE DAY...

INHALE

confidence,

EXHALE

doubt.

LESSON 1: WHAT TO DO NEXT

Objectives:

I. Understand the importance of establishing an exercise routine and schedule.

II. Understand that mild muscle soreness is an expected part of the process of getting stronger. In these cases, this is just weakness leaving your body!

To-Do:

Watch the "What To Do Next" video, take notes below as needed. ☐

LESSON 1: WHAT TO DO NEXT

Assignment:

As mentioned, it is so important to establish an exercise routine and schedule. What time of the day do you feel you have the most energy? Keep in mind, I recommend you wait at least 30 minutes after eating before engaging in physical activity and it is so important to stay hydrated. This is the time of day where you should aim to do this program and I encourage you to make this part of your daily routine - consistency is the key to success!
Be sure to look at my recommended weekly Exercise Schedule on page 147.

Reflect on your progress since you started this program and be proud of what you have achieved so far. Write down the improvements you notice about yourself physically, mentally, and emotionally. Then write down any goals you have for yourself moving forward with the program. Again, great job and keep up the good work!

Please write your response below.

LESSON 2: INTRODUCTION TO THE EXERCISE SCHEDULE

Objective:

I. Understand the importance of creating an **Exercise Schedule** that you can stick to.

To-Do:

- [ ] Watch the "Introduction to the Exercise Schedule" video, take notes below as needed.

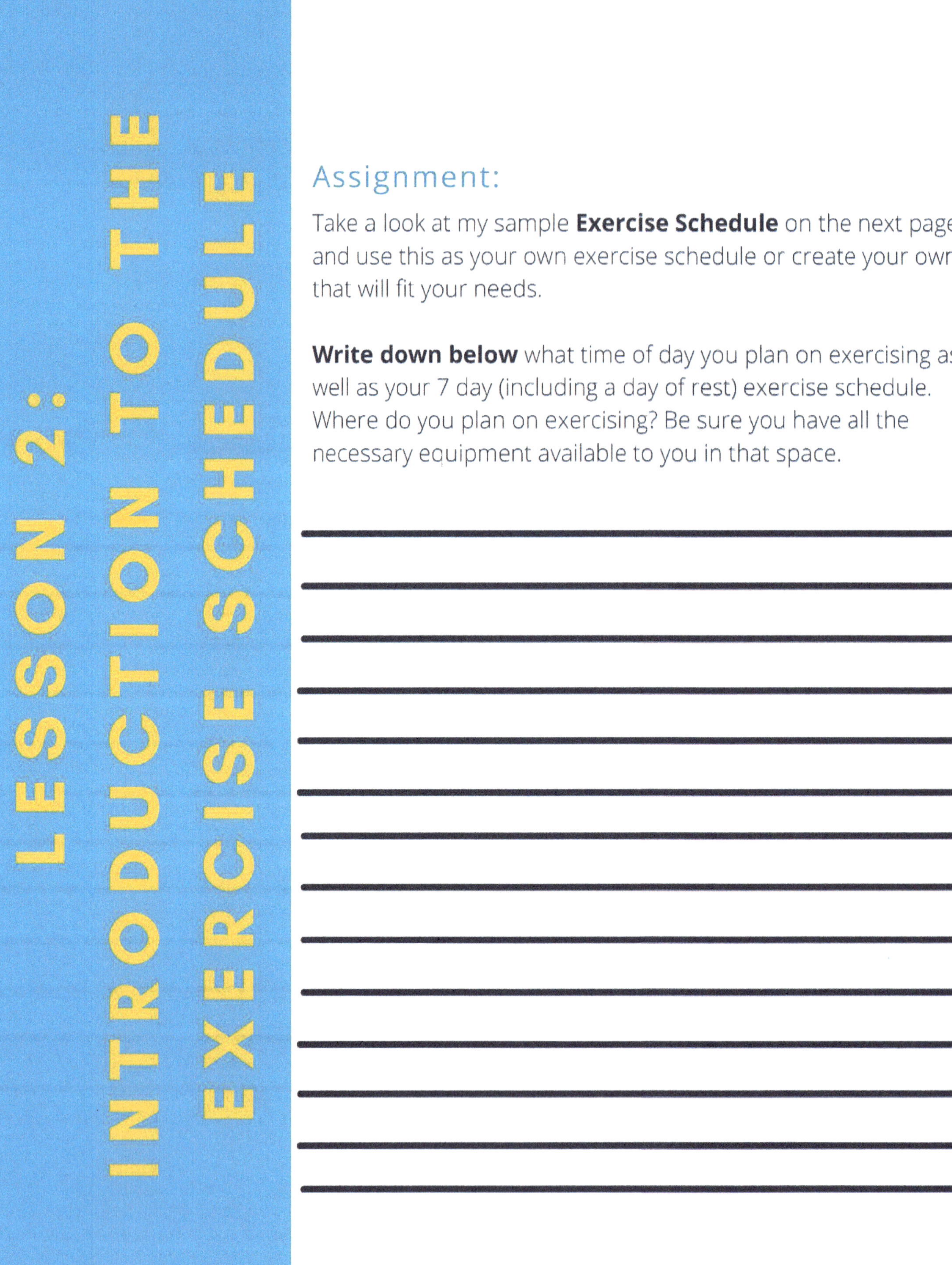

LESSON 2: INTRODUCTION TO THE EXERCISE SCHEDULE

Assignment:

Take a look at my sample **Exercise Schedule** on the next page and use this as your own exercise schedule or create your own that will fit your needs.

Write down below what time of day you plan on exercising as well as your 7 day (including a day of rest) exercise schedule. Where do you plan on exercising? Be sure you have all the necessary equipment available to you in that space.

LESSON 2: INTRODUCTION TO THE EXERCISE SCHEDULE

*If using my sample **Exercise Schedule** below, I encourage you to print it out and keep it in the area you plan on exercising in. If using your own schedule, be sure to do the same.*

	Monday	Tuesday	Wednesday	Thursday	Friday	Saturday	Sunday
Week 1	UPPER BODY WALKING	LOWER BODY WALKING	UPPER BODY	LOWER BODY WALKING	UPPER BODY WALKING	WALKING	REST
Week 2	LOWER BODY WALKING	UPPER BODY WALKING	LOWER BODY	UPPER BODY WALKING	LOWER BODY WALKING	WALKING	REST
Week 3	UPPER BODY WALKING	LOWER BODY WALKING	UPPER BODY	LOWER BODY WALKING	UPPER BODY WALKING	WALKING	REST
Week 4	LOWER BODY WALKING	UPPER BODY WALKING	LOWER BODY	UPPER BODY WALKING	LOWER BODY WALKING	WALKING	REST
Week 5	UPPER BODY WALKING	LOWER BODY WALKING	UPPER BODY	LOWER BODY WALKING	UPPER BODY WALKING	WALKING	REST
Week 6	LOWER BODY WALKING	UPPER BODY WALKING	LOWER BODY	UPPER BODY WALKING	LOWER BODY WALKING	WALKING	REST

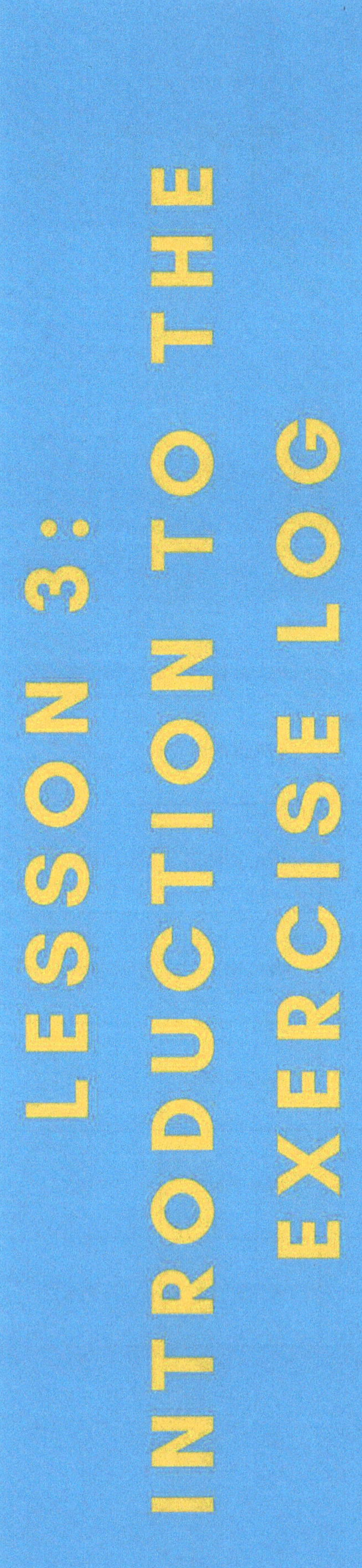

Objective:

I. Understand when to use the **Exercise Log** in this program.

II. Understand the importance of recording your exercise to help with accountability and to track your progress.

To-Do:

- [ ] Watch the "Introduction to the Exercise Log" video, take notes below as needed.

Assignment:

Please print and fill out the **Exercise Log** on the next page accordingly after exercising.

LESSON 3: INTRODUCTION TO THE EXERCISE LOG

Date	Time	Upper Body Exercises	Lower Body Exercises	Walking	Aerobic/Other

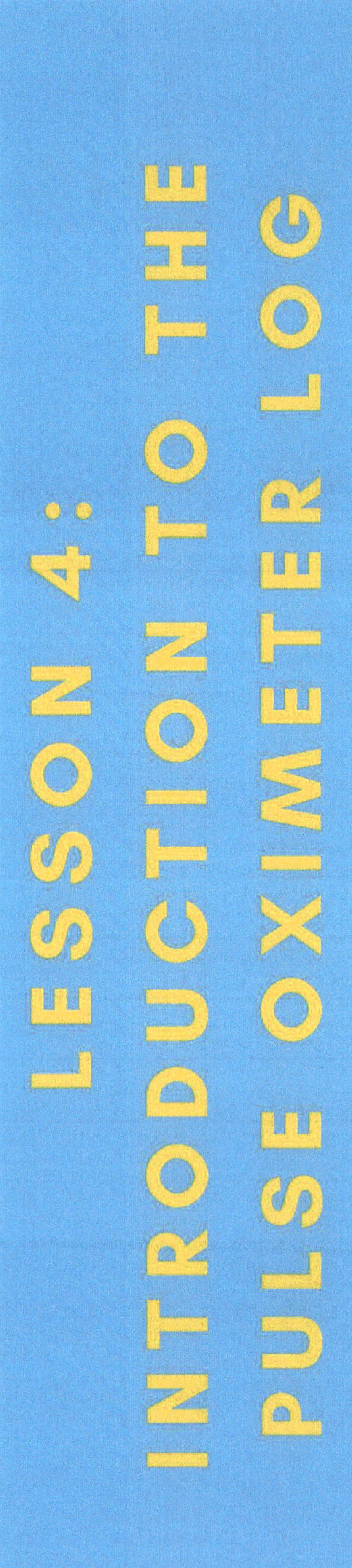
LESSON 4:
INTRODUCTION TO THE
PULSE OXIMETER LOG

Objective:

I. Understand when to use the **Pulse Oximeter Log** in this program.

II. Understand the importance of recording your exercise to help with accountability and to track your progress.

To-Do:

Watch the "Introduction to the Pulse Oximeter Log" video, take notes below as needed. ☐

Assignment:

Please print and fill out the **Pulse Oximeter Log** on the next page accordingly during **and** after exercising.

Please circle any oxygen saturation ***below 92%***!

LESSON 4: INTRODUCTION TO THE PULSE OXIMETER LOG

Please circle any oxygen saturation below 92%.

Date	Time	Lowest Oxygen Saturation (%)	Highest Heart Rate (bpm)	Oxygen (L) or Room Air	Activity What were you doing?	Weather Temperature, humidity, etc.

LESSON 5: INTRODUCTION TO THE WALKING LOG

Objective:

I. Understand when to use the **Walking Log** in this program.

II. Understand the importance of recording your exercise to help with accountability and to track your progress.

To-Do:

- [ ] Watch the "Introduction to the Walking Log" video, take notes below as needed.

Assignment:

Please print and fill out the Walking Log on the next page accordingly **before, during, AND after walking.**

Please circle any oxygen saturation ***below 92%!***

LESSON 5: INTRODUCTION TO THE WALKING LOG

Please circle any oxygen saturation <u>below 92%</u>.

Date	Distance (miles)	Flat or hills?	Time (min)	Number of Rests	Oxygen Saturation (%)	Heart Rate (bpm)	Oxygen (L) or Room Air
					Pre: During: After:	Pre: During: After:	Pre: During: After:
					Pre: During: After:	Pre: During: After:	Pre: During: After:
					Pre: During: After:	Pre: During: After:	Pre: During: After:
					Pre: During: After:	Pre: During: After:	Pre: During: After:
					Pre: During: After:	Pre: During: After:	Pre: During: After:

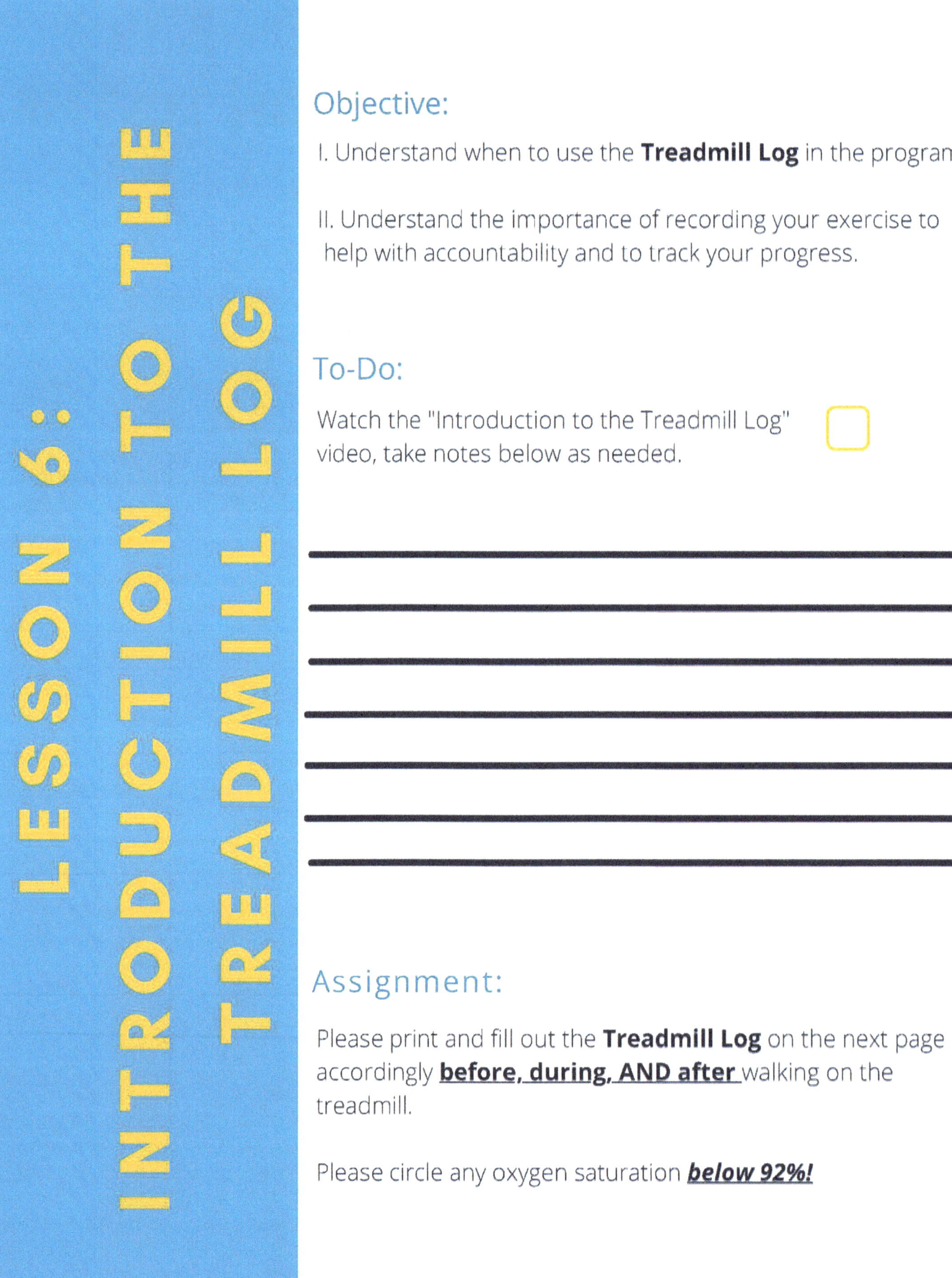

LESSON 6: INTRODUCTION TO THE TREADMILL LOG

Objective:

I. Understand when to use the **Treadmill Log** in the program.

II. Understand the importance of recording your exercise to help with accountability and to track your progress.

To-Do:

Watch the "Introduction to the Treadmill Log" video, take notes below as needed. ☐

Assignment:

Please print and fill out the **Treadmill Log** on the next page accordingly **<u>before, during, AND after</u>** walking on the treadmill.

Please circle any oxygen saturation ***<u>below 92%!</u>***

LESSON 6: INTRODUCTION TO THE TREADMILL LOG

Please circle any oxygen saturation <u>below 92%</u>.

Date	Speed (mph)	Incline (%)	Incline (min)	Distance (miles)	Time (min)	# of rests	Oxygen Saturation (%)	Heart Rate (bpm)	Oxygen (L) or Room Air
							Pre: During: After:	Pre: During: After:	Pre: During: After:
							Pre: During: After:	Pre: During: After:	Pre: During: After:
							Pre: During: After:	Pre: During: After:	Pre: During: After:
							Pre: During: After:	Pre: During: After:	Pre: During: After:
							Pre: During: After:	Pre: During: After:	Pre: During: After:

Conclusion

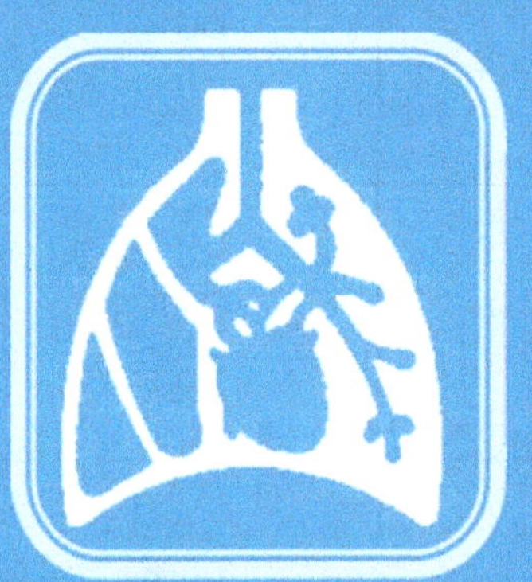

Congratulations!

To-Do:

Watch the "Congratulations!" video. ☐

You did it! Congratulations on completing the **Comprehensive Course!**

Be sure to print out your diploma and I encourage you to go back through this course frequently - it is a lot of information and may be beneficial to have a second look. From here, stick to your exercise schedule and reference this course as needed moving forward.

Don't forget to take the end-of-course survey.
We value your feedback!

Made in United States
North Haven, CT
08 February 2025

65500666R00091